SHEILA LAMB

This is Pregnancy After Infertility and Loss

Real-life experiences from the finally pregnant community

Thank you Pippa
much love
Sheila x

First edition

ISBN: 978-1-9993035-8-7

Cover art by Sheila Alexander
Editing by Sherron Mayes
Illustration by Sheila Alexander
Illustration by Phillip Reed

This book was professionally typeset on Reedsy.
Find out more at reedsy.com

Dedicated to all the incredibly strong women and men who became part of the finally pregnant community

Contents

Foreword

"But where is the support for this stage of our journey?"

This was the question I repeatedly asked when I became finally pregnant in 2018. At the time there wasn't any information or support, which is why I created the 'Finally Pregnant' Podcast. A few years later, and I'm so pleased to see how things have changed. Indeed, this very book by Sheila Lamb is one of those incredible pieces of support. It will help so many who may find themselves in the midst of complex emotions that can come with being pregnant after infertility and loss.

When we're trying to conceive, we often can't allow ourselves to think any further than a potential positive pregnancy test. That is our primary aim, our holy grail. And yes, finding out we are *actually* pregnant comes with an immediate and overwhelming joy comparable to little else. But then, in my own experience and of those who have shared their stories for Sheila's book, that joy can all too often be pushed swiftly aside, replaced by crippling anxiety and fear; "But what if it all goes wrong?"

Finding ourselves in the very position we have wanted to be in for months, years, decades even, but struggling to enjoy it, can be a difficult pill to swallow. We might feel ungrateful or that we don't deserve it. These are sentiments you'll find in the following stories. But, as you will also read from those who've shared their own experience, it is absolutely possible to be grateful beyond words whilst also finding being pregnant a struggle. If pregnancy hormones aren't enough, being pregnant after infertility and loss can conjure up a myriad more emotions.

Some of those reasons you'll read about include:

- Ongoing bleeding throughout pregnancy adding to the constant worry that something is going wrong. Many share of the fear of going to the toilet and seeing blood, but for some, that is a reality for weeks if not months, even for healthy pregnancies.
- The desire for morning sickness or other pregnancy symptom to offer validation that all's well, especially in the early days.
- The reality that is 'scanxiety'. Followed by the outpouring of relief on being told all is well, and perhaps even being lucky enough to hear that treasured sound of our miracle's heartbeat.
- You'll hear about milestones of past losses needing to be reached before feeling safe.
- The grief surrounding pregnancies that come after little ones lost. The bitter sweet feelings of seeing babies wearing clothes their older siblings never got to.

There is also a tendency for misunderstanding from those outside our community. Our well-meaning friends and family who genuinely think that being pregnant means we're 'fixed' when we feel anything but. We tentatively share our news to be met with sincere excitement that can be more than disconcerting given our journey – "Don't get too excited!" we say, not wanting to let them down if it all goes wrong.

As you'll read, there is so much more to say about the impact our journey may have on our subsequent parenting, pregnancy and parenting through a pandemic, surrogacy, donation, the pull to do it all over again for a sibling. Or choosing not to. The stories Sheila has curated do that so eloquently that I won't keep you from them too much longer.

Just to say that being finally pregnant is a precious place to find yourself, but please, as I hope you have during your trying to conceive journey, maintain a support network. Do things in your own time and, whilst we will likely never eradicate the anxiety altogether, do try to snatch back moments of joy wherever you can.

This is Pregnancy After Infertility and Loss – the true reality of being finally pregnant: scary and complex, but so wonderful.

Cat Strawbridge
   Host of the 'Finally Pregnant' Podcast.
   Socials @finallypregnant and @tryingyears.
   Website **www.catstrawbridge.com**

Acknowledgements

This book, and the 'Fertility Books' series it is part of, would not exist if it wasn't for the women and men who are part of the most amazing and supportive global community that ever existed. It wasn't until I joined Instagram after publishing my first book in 2018: *My Fertility Book – All the Fertility and Infertility Explanations you will ever need, from A to Z*, that I realised what 'community' really means. Although my roller-coaster infertility and loss journey ended happily several years ago, it has helped me to accept the emotions that come with all areas of infertility and loss, and are still part of me.

My thanks, firstly, go to my miracle, rainbow daughter Jessica, (a rainbow baby is one who's born after a loss). She means the world to me and is my reason for writing in order to help and support the trying to conceive community. Secondly, each contributor saw my vision for this series and has kindly shared their experience to support you. I appreciate each and every one of them, especially as we've never met in real life.

So in alphabetical order: Alex Kornswiet @ourbeautifulsurprise, Alyssa @healthyivf, Annette Pearson @thatwarriorannette, Arden Cartrette @themiscarriagedoula, Christina Oberon @xtina.o__, Clare @iwannabemamabear, Crystal-Gayle @4damani, Erin Bulcao @mybeautifulblunder, Grace Miano

@thegracemiano, Helena Tubridy @helenatubridy, Jasmine @glowful.path, Jennifer Roberston @msjenniferrobertson, Karen Hanson @aurafertility, Karen P, Kate Knapton @joji-iandco, Katy Jenkins @ivf_got_this_uk, Laura @Fertili_arty, Leah Irby @leahirby, Lianne Baker, Lyndsey Clabby @my-mindbodybaby, Mark @bombprooffamily, @me_becomes_we, Nora @thislimboland, Suzanne Minnis @the_baby_gaim and Tori Day @toridaywarrior.

If you would like to connect with any of these lovely people, there's a 'Resources' section at the back of this book.

The book cover illustration was by the author of *IF: A Memoir of Infertility*, Sheila Alexander, who was so supportive and patient as I stumbled to explain what I wanted for the book series. We both very much hope you relate to the couple as we follow them on their path to parenthood, and with the woman on the front of this cover looking at her scan photo. You'll find further illustrations by Sheila with some of the contributions. For more information visit her website: www.sheilaalexanderart.com or follow her on Instagram @sheilaalexanderart.

Like the other books in the series, I've included some illustrations in the hope that you can relate to them as much as the stories. Illustrator and author, Phillip Reed, created the illustrations for *My Fertility Book, Infertility Doesn't Care About Ethnicity* and for the other books in the series. He can be contacted on philr@live.co.uk and Instagram @the_phillustrator.

I'd also like to thank the following people who have encouraged and supported me to put my *Fertility Books* series together: my parents John and Freda (my Mum sadly passed away before this book was published), Judy Marell, Michelle Starkey, Jackie Chidwick, Claudia Sievers, Angie Conlon, Maria Bagao, Melissa Werry and Sue Monaghan.

Introduction

I'm delighted you're finally pregnant, but I'm sorry if you're struggling to feel the excitement you deserve. It's confusing, isn't it? You know you're fortunate, but at the same time, you're scared, unable to stop the 'What ifs?' bombarding you. I've been there too. It may have been a few years ago, but I so often see women on social media sharing the same emotions.

I couldn't understand why after six years of unexplained infertility – an unsuccessful Intra-Uterine Insemination (IUI) and In-Vitro Fertilisation (IVF) cycle, and an early pregnancy loss after egg donor IVF, I wasn't relaxing on cloud nine whilst browsing Mother and Baby magazines and making newborn purchases. We delayed sorting out the pushchair/car seat combo and decorating the nursery until my waters broke! Not exactly but it wasn't far off!! We barely took any photos of my bump, and there were none with my husband and I, except for a photo shoot a few weeks before my due date. We didn't sign up for any birthing classes – I'd previously trained as a midwife so that may have had something to do with it, but it's different when you're the one giving birth! That's how we protected ourselves, scared our happiness would be ripped away. Luckily that pregnancy was successful, and our treasured little girl is growing up to be the most gorgeous, funny, kind daughter I could ever have wished for. But then I'm biased!

In hindsight, I wish I'd enjoyed my one and only pregnancy a little more. And that's why I contacted so many amazing women from social media to bring together their experiences. It's the fifth book in my *Fertility Books* series – each edition a collection of testimonies from parents who've experienced the struggle to bring their baby home.

They saw my vision for this book – that none of us wants anyone to feel alone on their challenging journey to parenthood. It's not easy to share such personal information and it's hard to put it into words. But they bravely share their emotions honestly, such as what helped or didn't help them, practical advice for keeping calm, and how they're supporting others in the infertility community. They also want their stories to open up the narrative in society about finally being pregnant after infertility and loss, because a woman, especially, is very vulnerable at this time.

Some women don't announce their pregnancy until they're halfway through gestation, and that's OK. They have their reasons. There's an ingrained expectation that you shouldn't announce your pregnancy until the twelfth week, because you won't lose a baby after that time. Sadly, many people know differently. In my case, I told family and friends immediately, because when we'd had a miscarriage, we felt there was a lack of empathy from some – so I wanted everyone to experience the joy of our pregnancy this time, in case we needed support. How you handle your announcement is right for you.

At some point, your nearest and dearest will know that you're pregnant even though you may still have fears. If you can't express why you're not full of joy, or why you're suddenly tearful or why you don't want them buying baby clothes, yet ... maybe hand over this book and leave them alone while you make them a cuppa.

I also hope this book, and my book series, helps others who haven't gone through the struggle to get pregnant and bring their baby home – such as family, friends, hospital staff, and other healthcare professionals – to better understand what it's like for those who have.

As the well-known author CS Lewis once said (or maybe wrote): "We read to know we are not alone. Reading is that journey of finding people who feel the same way". This is what I hope you feel after reading *This is Pregnancy After Infertility and Loss*.

Wishing you the very best
  Sheila xx

Letter to someone who's finally pregnant

Dear Friend,

May I offer my congratulations to you? I know you've been through so much to finally become pregnant, and I know you can't let your guard down. Not yet, anyway. You want to protect your heart just in case... You're frightened to get your hopes up, just in case... You don't feel like celebrating, just in case... When it's been a huge struggle to conceive, there's long-lasting trauma that doesn't end with a positive pregnancy test.

I really do understand, and so do the women who've shared their stories in this book. Everyone is unique, yet, finally seeing those two lines after infertility, unsuccessful fertility treatment, pregnancy, or baby loss, means the emotions you're experiencing now you're finally pregnant, are the same as ours. This is normal. And it's OK to feel this way. It can feel a little like survivor's guilt, can't it? Why am I pregnant when so many women are still trying? But you were one of those women still trying, and someone else was where you are now. It's your turn now and you aren't ungrateful.

As with my other books in the *Fertility Series,* I contacted women who've dealt with infertility and loss, as well as those who've eventually had successful pregnancies. They all said a big, fat, "Yes!" keen to help others and share their experiences. Finally being pregnant brings a new set of emotions that aren't necessarily what you expected. And if this is your first-ever positive pregnancy test after, perhaps, years of unsuccessful fertility treatments, you're like a deer caught in the headlights experiencing utter shock. We know how that feels.

When you're trying to get pregnant, you can't help but imagine how it will be when it happens. You've spent many months and quite possibly years, dreaming about this moment, wondering how you'll feel, what you'll say to people – but like many long-held dreams, the reality can be very different. Please, don't be hard on yourself. This is unknown territory. And there isn't a 'How to feel' manual with a right or wrong way. Hopefully, the testimonies in this book will ensure you feel validated and not alone, which is so very important on this roller-coaster journey.

You'll read that pregnancy after loss is complicated:

- distinguishing between how you WANT to feel, how you think you SHOULD feel, and how you REALLY feel
- convincing yourself that you can only enjoy the pregnancy once you've reached certain milestones
- being terrified this pregnancy will end the same way as previous ones, and feeling guilty for those thoughts
- learning to enjoy your pregnancy and making it a magical experience by having a supportive birth team.

As you can see from the above, finally being pregnant isn't easy, but it can be enjoyable, even if you don't think so right now. You may also feel contradictory emotions, i.e; worried but excited; sad but happy. And that's OK.

A lot of newly pregnant women experience awkwardness around their friends who are still struggling, whether in their social circle or online. Again, that's a common feeling and it's because you empathise, having walked in their shoes. They're likely excited for you even if they feel sad for themselves – a seesaw of emotions you'll be familiar with. You'll know the best way to move forward because it'll be how you'd like to be treated. And I bet they'd be the first to tell you to enjoy being pregnant.

If you've spent a long time in the uber-supportive TTC and/or loss community, then it's not uncommon to feel you don't fit in with other ante/pre-natal women. You may think you're the only one who's had a struggle, that all these other women just looked at their partners and fell pregnant. But one in eight couples worldwide experience infertility, and it's estimated that in the UK, one in four pregnancies end in loss during pregnancy or birth*. So, the chances are that if there are more than eight women in your pregnancy yoga class, you're not alone.

If you underwent fertility treatment, you may remember sitting in the clinic waiting room and trying not to lock eyes with another woman. Yet also feeling desperate to speak with them. What if another woman in your yoga class feels just like you? I told two of the women at my yoga class of only five women that my baby was an IVF baby, conceived with a donor egg. And do you know what – one lady who was expecting her second baby had IVF to conceive her first! I wasn't alone.

Sadly, you won't always meet an empathetic healthcare worker now that you're pregnant. Some simply won't understand why you're so anxious, why you want a scan when a scan isn't due, and why, when you do have a scan, you immediately say with a catch in your voice, "I've had a miscarriage before." There are 'pregnancy after loss' stickers available that can be put on your notes so that midwives, doctors etc are aware, and will hopefully understand why your anxiety levels are sky-high and choose their words more carefully.

Parenting after infertility and loss can also bring up more conflicting emotions – such as feeling you can't complain about your kids because there-are-so-many-people-who-can't-have-kids-so-you-need-to-be-more-grateful. You're only human, of course you're going to be exhausted, scramble to put on clean clothes, and hate that you haven't washed your hair in so long you can't remember. That's the reality of parenthood, and just because you've struggled or have children who are no longer with you earthside, this new baby is unique, and people won't necessarily understand what you've been through. You can be ever so grateful, but also vent.

Because you're used to challenging issues on your journey to parenthood, even when you have your healthy baby safely in your arms, you still might feel scared that something awful might happen. The times I woke my sleeping baby up because I thought she'd stopped breathing you wouldn't believe! Having dreams that you can't find your baby/child or that they've been taken from you is also common. This still happens to me and

7

my daughter's eleven! But it isn't as often and to be honest, I probably should have spoken to someone about these thoughts a long time ago. I'm just trying to reassure you that it isn't just you.

Finally, I just want to say that 'You. Are. Pregnant.' Digest that. Against all the odds, you're expecting a baby. This may be the furthest into a pregnancy you've ever been. It's fan-dabby-doozy! Celebrate the small wins. Take one day at a time. And remember, you're not alone, Mama.

Much love,
   Sheila and the contributors xx

*Taken from Tommy's charity (UK) 2022

Letter to someone who hasn't been through infertility and loss

Dear Friend,

Thank you for opening this book and wanting to learn more about pregnancy after infertility and loss. It affects more people than you probably realise; there are approximately twenty-three million miscarriages every year worldwide*, and approximately one in eight couples, or as high as one in five couples in the US** experience infertility. I'd hazard a guess that you know someone who's one of these statistics, even though they may not have shared that with you.

You may be slightly confused why a woman whose been trying for years to get and stay pregnant – and is finally pregnant – would feel different to someone who conceived straight away. It's complicated if you haven't experienced it.

When a woman conceives easily, she'll assume she'll give birth after nine months, and during that time there will be some sickness, feeling tired, along with regular appointments to check everything's going well. She may also go to birth preparation classes with a partner, if she has one. All the delightful, happy events one expects to happen during pregnancy and is often portrayed in TV series and films.

When a woman has been trying to conceive for many months or years, and only knows disappointment after disappointment, especially following unsuccessful fertility treatments, such as In-Vitro Fertilisation – it isn't unusual to do more than three rounds – her only experience is one of devastation. When a woman loses her baby during the pregnancy however she conceives, the next time she's pregnant, she may assume she'll lose the baby fearing the same thing will happen again.

Here's an analogy that might help: are you scared of something, say a dog, because you were once bitten or chased, and ever since then, all dogs put the fear of God into you? No matter how many people tell you it won't happen again, that it's a different breed of dog, this dog is nice, you have a fear of the same outcome. Multiply your feelings a million times, and that's how it feels for someone who's had problems conceiving, or had a loss during pregnancy.

Believe it or not, the woman and their partner, if there is one, are traumatised by what they've been through ... just like the person who's always scared of dogs. And that's compounded because society doesn't talk about infertility, miscarriage, and baby loss. And when a woman is finally pregnant and feels anxious seeing a positive pregnancy test, scared that those nine months won't end with a baby, she may keep those feelings to herself.

Over eight million children have been born since the first UK IVF baby in 1978. Around 2.5 million IVF cycles are carried out every year and this number increases, around the world, every year. The mother of the first IVF baby had blocked Fallopian tubes, and therefore, the egg and the sperm were unlikely to meet whilst she tried to fall pregnant naturally, regardless as to whether she relaxed or put her legs in the air after intercourse, or prayed harder. IVF is now used for a variety of medical conditions – note the word 'medical' – such as Endometriosis, Polycystic Ovarian Syndrome, early menopause, and male factor issues, but for many others, there's no known medical cause.

Sadly, though, IVF doesn't always guarantee a baby. IVF cycles can be cancelled at any point before transferring an embryo, which is devastating. The chances of being successful through this fertility treatment will depend on the age of the woman's eggs and other factors relevant to the woman and her partner. But on average, only thirty-seven per cent of IVF cycles for women under thirty-five result in a baby, which means sixty-three per cent aren't successful.

IVF isn't entered into lightly; it takes a strong person/couple to get through the demands, not only on the woman's body, but with fitting the regular appointments/treatments into their lives. And often, it's a busy woman who has to find the time, sometimes in secret from family and friends, to do most, if not all of the following:

- hours and hours of medical research – trawling websites, reading books and articles, listening to podcasts, interacting on Facebook groups, and watching YouTube videos
- researching the best nutritional supplements for herself and her partner

- researching toxins in the house that could be affecting her/their fertility, then throwing those items away and replacing them with safe beauty/bathing/household products
- navigating medical insurance forms if applicable
- reading and replying to emails, taking and making phone calls with fertility clinic staff
- diarising appointments for investigations, scans, blood tests, for her and her partner
- ordering medications and recording dosage along with the exact times they're to be taken
- giving herself injections (or her partner/a friend may do this), to increase the number of eggs she produces and taking other medications to thicken her womb lining and help the embryo implant
- dealing emotionally with family and friend's pregnancy announcements, gender reveals, baby showers and birth announcements
- ensuring she's carrying out daily or at least regular self-care for herself – journaling, meditation, exercise, mindfulness etc
- possibly attending alternative therapy appointments such as acupuncture, reiki, reflexology, Emotional Freedom Technique (EFT), yoga
- may have sessions with a fertility counsellor or coach
- looking for local support groups
- if doing treatment overseas, researching flights, accommodation, and organising currency.

Phew! And breathe! Quite a list on top of living a 'normal' life, isn't it?

If you don't know much about pregnancy and loss, there are many 'losses' between a positive test and birth:

- a positive home pregnancy test that was short-lived and became a 'chemical pregnancy', blighted ovum, missed miscarriage, ectopic pregnancy, or early miscarriage – the woman or couple experienced the excitement of seeing a positive result only to have it snatched away days or a few weeks later.
- a 'vanishing twin' – at the first scan, two pregnancy sacs are seen revealing twins! But at the following scan, there's only one baby and the woman hasn't experienced any bleeding or cramps to indicate she's lost one of the twins. That's heart-breaking, despite still being pregnant with one baby.
- molar pregnancy is when there's a chromosomal abnormality that occurs at the time of fertilisation – it's usually discovered during the twelve-week ultrasound scan when the heartbeat can't be seen, and the placenta is abnormal. There's a risk the woman will develop choriocarcinoma and require chemotherapy. She now grieves the loss of her baby whilst dealing with the reality that the pregnancy endangered her life.
- termination for medical reasons (TFMR), compassionate induction or medically-based termination is when a much-wanted baby has a fatal or life-limiting condition, and the parent(s) decide to end the pregnancy. It's a tremendously difficult decision for parents to make and they experience significant grief and sadness.
- a late miscarriage happens between fourteen and twenty-four weeks of pregnancy in the UK, or twenty weeks in other countries – the parent(s) have seen their baby developing

on their ultrasound, have a scanned image and maybe a 3D photo, and have shared the exciting news with family and friends, so the loss is experienced by everyone.

· stillbirth is when the baby dies in the womb before birth – in the UK after twenty-four weeks and in the US after twenty weeks of pregnancy. The loss of a baby this late into the pregnancy brings unimaginable pain; the mother usually gives birth rather than has a caesarean (which is a major operation), and sometimes days after she has found out she has lost the baby.

At four weeks pregnant when most women/couples see a positive pregnancy test, cells are creating the baby's brain. At six weeks the baby's heartbeat can be seen and heard on a vaginal ultrasound scan. At seven weeks, they can make jerky movements, and by twelve weeks you can tell if they're a boy or a girl.

Maybe now you're beginning to see how finally being pregnant after infertility and loss isn't plain sailing. To help navigate these choppy waters, reading other people's stories can be so supportive. It helps the woman to not feel alone and validates her feelings, which is so important for how she'll get through the next part of her journey to motherhood. You can help her by simply listening. Read the stories in this book – the women who've shared theirs know how important it is to find others who've felt the same, and they'll help you to support your loved one in the best way.

If you're a healthcare worker, midwife, or working in an ante/pre-natal dept, please take the time to research what's involved in IVF – for example, what medications the woman may still be on and why, and learn about all the different pregnancy losses, as this will help you understand why she's so anxious now she's finally pregnant. My guidance to birth educators, yoga teachers, the National Childbirth Trust (UK) and other charities etc who support pregnant women – please ensure your marketing materials don't contain triggers for women who've struggled. And don't assume everyone has conceived naturally; remember the stats mentioned earlier.

If you work with women in the post-natal period; if you know the woman has struggled to take her baby home, understand that her emotions are more complex and that she's at a higher risk of developing postnatal depression (PND). Give them time to talk about their journey, even if you've heard it already. Above all, please, don't judge them or ever start a sentence with "At least..."

Pregnancy is an amazing experience, one that should be enjoyed and cherished. With your understanding and support, you can help so many women who are finally pregnant after infertility and loss.

Much love,

Sheila & the contributor's xx

*From Tommy's charity (UK)
**From Centers for Disease Control and Prevention

It's complicated

I was just a woman, standing in front of a home pregnancy test, praying for it to be positive.

I remember that moment like it was yesterday. My heart beating faster and faster, impatiently waiting the three minutes which felt like a lifetime, squinting to see a second line. Then I'd put the stick down and walk away, trying to distract myself, only to be drawn back in anticipation. My palms were sweaty and for the first time in a long while, I allowed myself to picture my growing belly and holding another baby in my arms. The alarm on the timer woke me from my daydream. I grabbed the magic stick that had become a source of heartbreak over the last six years and took a deep breath ...

TWO LINES! TWO FREAKING LINES! Three pregnancy tests later and it finally started to sink in. The excitement was off the charts as if I'd just jumped out of an aeroplane and were free-falling through the air. It was exhilarating. For a moment. Until I realized that we'd jumped out of that plane six months ago and face-planted on the ground.

Our path to get here had been filled with heartbreak and hope.

You can read my entire story in my book, *The Injustice of Infertility*. However, I'll give you the short version so you understand why the joy turned into fear.

Six years earlier, when my husband and I got married, we immediately tried for a baby on our honeymoon. Like anyone else, we were unprepared for the struggles that came our way. After six months we saw a fertility specialist who recommended IVF, given my husband's sperm quality and my irregular cycle. Halfway through the first cycle, they discovered that the lining on my uterus wouldn't thicken. Over the next year, I was subjected to multiple exploratory surgeries, hormone replacement therapies and anything else you can think of, including Viagra pessaries. On top of that, we tried a whole range of natural therapies, different diets, and acupuncture. But nothing worked. Eventually, our fertility specialist advised that the only way we were going to have a baby of our own was via a surrogate.

Fortunately, my sister-in-law volunteered to have a baby for us. But that wasn't the end. Our surrogacy journey lasted two years, included nine IVF cycles, and one miscarriage finally leading us to a healthy baby boy, Luca.

Two weeks after Luca was born, I discovered I was pregnant again. Me. Pregnant. WTF! Unfortunately, at our nine-week ultrasound, I heard the words you never want to hear – *I'm sorry, there's no heartbeat.* THAT WAS WHEN I HIT ROCK BOTTOM. The injustice and devastation made me numb and angry. SO ANGRY.

And here I was, six months later with the trauma and grief

behind me, but still very present. I was emotionally and physically exhausted. And at that moment, with that stick held tightly in my sweaty hand, it all came flooding back.

When I think of pregnancy after loss, the phrase that comes to mind is 'It's complicated'. I wanted to be pregnant more than anything in this world, but I was dreading the path in front of me. I yearned to celebrate and feel excitement and joy, but instead, I was consumed by fear and kept waiting for the pain and disappointment that usually ensued. I couldn't distinguish between how I WANTED to feel, how I SHOULD feel, and how I REALLY felt. It was a constant struggle.

The wait between peeing on that stick, getting our blood results, and the twelve-week scan was pure agony. We were living in limbo yet again. Our future was uncertain. The two-week wait had been replaced by a twelve-week wait. My morning sickness was a mixture of dread and relief. On the days I felt well, there was no relief – my mind always jumped to the worst-case scenario. In my last pregnancy, I knew something wasn't right when my boobs stopped hurting. While they hurt, I knew I was pregnant. I was constantly squeezing them to make sure I was still pregnant which must have looked very weird for those around me. Each trip to the bathroom was met with fear. Would this be the morning I'd see blood? Every wipe I'd hold my breath and pray for the best.

By the time I went for our first ultrasound, I felt like a crazy woman. Walking into our appointment was terrifying. The last time we were in that very same room, it didn't end well. And that replayed over and over in my mind.

But we made it, and we heard that magic noise. *Gadoook, Gadoonk, Gadoonk.* Even today, hearing that sound fills me with tears of relief.

We didn't tell anyone we were pregnant until after that scan – even our parents. We'd dragged them along on this roller-coaster for such a long time. They'd all been through too much disappointment, and we didn't want to do it to them AGAIN. So, the phone call to finally tell our family was filled with relief and fear. We tried to manage their, and our expectations by saying things like, "We'll see how things go" and "Let's try not to get too ahead of ourselves".

Apart from our family, there were very few people we told until it was too obvious that I couldn't hide it any longer. We didn't want to jinx it. I thought if I put it out there, and opened my heart a little, the other shoe would drop. By then, I expected things to go wrong for us because that was the pattern our checkered seven-year fertility journey had followed. Plus, the shame of having to take back our pregnancy news and tell people if something went wrong, made me feel sick to my stomach.

I was shocked that I was still triggered by other people's pregnancy announcements despite being pregnant myself. I was jealous that other people had no fear of putting it out there, but I couldn't bring myself to announce my own. Out of all the people we knew, we were the ones who should have been shouting it from the rooftops, because it was a true miracle. After all, a board of doctors had labelled me infertile and told us this wasn't possible.

There was no big reveal or announcement, just quiet words in corridors and behind closed doors. We were 'quietly and cautiously hopeful'. And when we did tell people, their reaction made me feel worse – they were more excited than I was! I knew this was such a blessing and how many others would kill to be in our position, so I felt extremely selfish and ungrateful.

The time between scans was painfully long. And then at each scan, I'd spend the first part of the appointment holding my breath, just waiting to hear the heartbeat. By then I was thirty-eight, so my pregnancy was considered 'geriatric'. Whoever coined that term needs to be punched in the face! But because of that, I had extra appointments, which allowed my fear and uncertainty to subside a little each time.

At around twenty-four weeks, I had my glucose test for gestational diabetes. It came back positive and knocked me on my ass. I have no idea why it affected me so much, but I remember driving home after getting the test results with tears streaming down my face. I felt like a failure, and it allowed a little more doubt to creep back in. Over the last six months, I'd started to trust that my body knew what it was doing. But perhaps it didn't. I was old, infertile, and now I had gestational diabetes. Over the next three months, I monitored my diet, measured my blood glucose levels, and kept a diary. I was annoyed that I couldn't eat ice cream or indulge my pregnancy cravings. But it was a small price to pay.

Despite this being our second child, we went to the recommended birthing classes. Our last experience with birth was very different, given the fact that someone else was carrying our baby. We didn't need to know all that stuff back then. We were merely passengers. But now it was my body. At the classes, I remember looking around the room, wondering how hard these couples had to fight to get here. Was this easy for them? They spoke about baby names and the excitement of their upcoming arrival. I envied them a little.

We didn't have a baby shower or organize a pregnancy photo-shoot. On reflection, I have barely any pictures of me pregnant. We didn't decorate the nursery until the very end, and we only bought a baby capsule after our little girl arrived, and we were undecided on baby names. We were so focused on getting to the end and having our baby in our arms, that we missed the miracle of pregnancy. And that makes me sad.

At around thirty-six weeks our baby still hadn't turned around and her head was sitting right under my ribcage. Our doctor presented us with our options, and we had to make a decision. Do we risk turning her around so I could birth normally, or do we elect to have a caesarean? I was once again devastated.Nothing about our path to get here was normal, and I was desperate to experience childbirth. As weird as that sounds, I wasn't afraid of the pain, I simply wanted the maternal picture I had in my head of bringing a child into this world, naturally. But we decided the risk wasn't worth it, and a couple of weeks later our baby girl was born via emergency caesarean.

To be honest with you, I can't remember a lot about our pregnancy. It didn't make a lot of sense until I learned that stress can affect how memories are formed. People have a more difficult time creating short-term memories when stressed and turning them into long-term memories.

Today, as I watch our two babies sleeping soundly, I often reflect how our journey wasn't filled with joy, excitement, and fairy dust. But it was real and raw. Ours is a story packed with strength, triumph, courage, and determination.

For a long time afterwards, I punished myself feeling guilty for not being able to experience the joy and excitement everyone else seemed to feel.

But this is PREGNANCY AFTER LOSS. It's tough. Seeing those two lines on a stick doesn't mean, I was having a baby. It represented, instead, the beginning of yet another race to the finish line.

If you've gone through pregnancy loss and trauma to get here, there's a valid reason WHY you feel like this and why you can't open your heart to the possibilities of a healthy pregnancy. It's not that you're crazy, ungrateful or weak. IT'S COMPLICATED!

The important thing is that you know this is normal. You're not alone. It's OK to be angry that the joy of a 'safe' pregnancy has been stolen from you. You don't need to punish yourself for being more anxious than excited.

My journey through infertility, IVF, surrogacy, and pregnancy loss, inspired me to become a fertility coach. So, I've created a community for women who are pregnant after infertility or pregnancy loss. YOUR PREGNANCY HAVEN provides support, connection, inspiration, and information throughout your pregnancy – so you feel heard, validated, and relieved that you're not alone. So you can appreciate the joy of your pregnancy, rather than just chasing that finish line.

Jennifer Robertson @msjenniferrobertson

Ramblings in the morning

It's 1:39 a.m. and I'm wide awake for no reason at all, in the middle of the night. This is good. This always happens to me when I'm pregnant. It happened every single night of my last pregnancy. This is good. This is good.

And then I start coughing. I've had a horrible chest and head cold for over a week now and I find myself choking. I've been sleeping on the couch most nights so my husband can get some rest. Wait, I'm only awake because I'm choking, and I can't breathe? This isn't because I'm pregnant. Something's wrong. Something's wrong. I'm losing this pregnancy, aren't I? Oh, God. I can't do this again. I can't survive this again. I should take another test to reassure myself. But... what if the line on the pregnancy test is lighter? Oh my God. I can't. I can't.

I click on the TV and turn the volume down so my husband doesn't wake up as I decided to sleep in our marital bed last night. I scroll through Netflix and find a random episode of 'Family Guy'. I've seen every episode of this show about fifty times, so the sights and sounds are familiar and strangely comforting. I nibble on a few saltines (soda crackers) I keep next to my bed so I don't wake up nauseous. I'm then able to slowly drift back to sleep. I wake up before my alarm at 5:40 a.m.

I'm not nauseous. Why am I not nauseous? Is it because I ate those saltines? I probably didn't even need to eat them. I'm just fooling myself into thinking I'm nauseous. I was so sick last week, I thought I was dying. Why don't I feel that sick anymore? What's wrong? Something's wrong. Oh my God. I'm losing this pregnancy.

I force myself to get up. I brush my teeth. I avoid looking at my reflection in the mirror. I feel a pang of guilt as I use my facewash that has salicylic acid in it, resolving to head to the store later and buy a safer brand. I wander into the kitchen and eat a mandarin. It's delicious. So, I eat another one. And then I eat a third one. And then I giggle because it seems as if my embryos, named 'Linus' and 'Lucy' are big fans of citrus.

Stop thinking like that. You can't think like that. Why do you name all your embryos? Why do you make them seem so human when they're just little balls of cells that might have stopped growing? You're probably going to have a miscarriage. You're so stupid. You did this to yourself. This is what you get for letting yourself get attached.

A wave of nausea rolls over me. I swallow hard. Wait. Maybe... no. It's probably not morning sickness. It's just heartburn because I just smashed three mandarins in my face like an idiot. And I'm queasy because I keep coughing. That's definitely it.

I sit on the couch and wish I'd been able to see into the future when I decided to take this week off from work. I didn't think my cycle would work, so I figured I'd spend the week healing, Christmas shopping and drinking eggnog martinis while I put my Christmas decorations up. Instead, I find myself bawling on the couch thinking about my ultrasound on Thursday. I can't do this again. I can't live through another miscarriage. I can't see the funny look on the ultrasound tech's face and hear the weirdly detached words of my doctor. I can't feel that rush of indescribable rage when the doctor refers to my dying embryos as 'babies' because that makes them seem like they really are babies when they're just chunks of tissue with abnormal chromosomes. I'm a terrible mother. A good mother would never think like that. Maybe I don't deserve to be a mother. Maybe that's been the problem all along.

Now my head is aching, and my stomach is churning. I sneeze and feel a familiar tightness low in my belly. Great. I'm cramping. I'm probably going to bleed any second, although last time, I had severe pains before the bleeding started. Why do I keep comparing this pregnancy to the last one? I don't want them to be the same. I want this one to end with a baby in my arms, not with my heart torn to shreds as I'm being wheeled into the operating room for a D&C. Think positive. All signs are positive. Betas are through the roof. You're exhausted. You're sick. This is good. This is good.

Everything's going to be okay. I touch my belly. If I push hard enough, it feels sore. It's either the cyst on my ovary, or it's my uterus.

My hands are shaking and I'm dizzy. It's because you've been crying too hard. You need to calm down. I want to call my nurse and ask if I can come in for another beta today. I don't do it though. I don't want her to think that I'm weak. I don't want her to hear me cry.

What the hell is wrong with me? I'm hungry. Part of me wants another mandarin. Another part of me wants chicken fingers. Or hash browns. Or both. With lots of ketchup, which I normally hate. This is good. Right?

I'm so tired. I just don't know what to do or how to feel anymore. I don't want to feel anymore.

This is too hard. Three more days. Three more days until my ultrasound. Three more days until I'll know whether I can keep bawling or feel more hopeful. Three more days.

I can do this. I think.

Karen P

Admitting the feelings of jealousy even when finally pregnant

Being pregnant after miscarriage was easily one of the more difficult things that I'd been through. After the trauma of loss, the fear of losing another baby was consuming my every thought. When I saw another pregnant woman, I'd wonder if she ever felt this fear. Was her journey to motherhood simple and quick?

As a woman, I was raised to believe jealousy was a negative emotion. Feeling jealous of others may not be ideal but it's an emotion we can't help but experience from time to time. While I battled infertility, after each of my two miscarriages, I went through many stages of grief, and part of my grief was being envious of women who both got pregnant naturally and didn't know what it was like to lose a baby. For the longest time, I thought that emotion was something to feel ashamed of and I kept those feelings to myself. It wasn't until my pregnancy with our rainbow baby, Cameron, that I accepted that I was jealous, and that it was okay to feel like that.

When you've experienced a miscarriage, everything changes. Your ability to be happy for someone else is different than it was before. The joy that you feel for a family member or a friend may be expressed as jealousy, envy, sadness but that doesn't mean that you're a terrible person, even though it may feel like you are in the moment. What helped me the most was learning to own the fact that I was jealous. It was freeing to say the words aloud, *"I'm jealous of other pregnant women"*.

During my first trimester of pregnancy after miscarriage, I'd be so envious of any woman who was around fourteen-plus weeks pregnant. *"It must be nice to be in the 'safe zone,'"* I'd think to myself, knowing that there wasn't a safe zone. Once I finally entered the second trimester, I thought the jealousy would get easier to manage, but the truth is, there's always going to be something you want and don't have. Then when you are closer to full-term, every birth announcement stings because you so badly want to hold your rainbow baby in your arms. You want to know that they are breathing and okay, so you're jealous of every Mama on social media that announces the birth of their little ones. Especially those who were due after you.

Admitting that you are still jealous of others even after you are finally pregnant makes you human. It shows what you've been through is a part of your journey and it's nothing to feel ashamed of.

Arden Cartrette @themiscarriagedoula

I am loving every second of my pregnancy

I thought I'd hate being pregnant.

I thought that after so many losses – six miscarriages including one horrific ectopic – and so much pain, the door to celebrating being pregnant would be closed to me forever.

I thought I'd want to see the positive pregnancy test and then have the doctors hand me my baby and skip the whole pregnancy shebang!

I thought that pregnancy after infertility and loss was an impossible dream. I was wrong!

As I write this, I'm thirty-two weeks pregnant and loving every second, minus the acid reflux!

What I do not feel is a sense of impending doom every day and I no longer feel crippled by fear, and I honestly thought I would. In fact, I feel such a strong connection with my little one – another surprise as we used donor eggs and I was terrified about bonding, that I wouldn't feel she was mine – but she is one hundred per cent mine and I can honestly say there's no difference between using my own eggs to get pregnant rather than donor eggs. Without question, I was always meant to have her.

Since then, I've felt so much more positive about this pregnancy as there was a higher chance of it working. That was another worry to check off my list. And the list, my friend was long!

One thing my infertility journey has given me though is anxiety – bad, bad, bad anxiety. And I now tend to catastrophise... everything! I thought this would apply to the pregnancy itself but it honestly hasn't. I now love being pregnant, so much so, that I don't want it to end! Selfishly, I want my 'us' time, just me and my little girl kicking inside me to carry on. I adore seeing my body change as my little one grows, and boy, does she love it when I rub my tummy! I'm also going a little easier on myself with diet and exercise than when we were TTC.

Sure, I have the worst *scanxiety*, but there's nothing I can do to change what happens at those scans. It's out of my control, so worrying is a waste of my energy. So bad was my anxiety surrounding scans, especially in the first trimester, that I was having scans before my official scans to make sure everything was OK! I still don't love going to scans... until the sonographer tells me everything is OK, and then they are the best thing ever!

Sure, I still get worried when something doesn't feel right and I still dread seeing red when I go to the loo, but I don't let this control my every waking thought. So, if you're dreading being pregnant, scared of something going wrong as it has before, my

31

advice is don't be! Trust in your pregnancy and trust in your little one. Yes, there will be times when you'll feel anxious; I was too terrified to even go for a walk in my first trimester for fear of bringing on a miscarriage! But believe me, the good days far outnumber the bad ones. So, relax and enjoy. You'll be A-Okay sister!

Clare @iwannabeamamabear

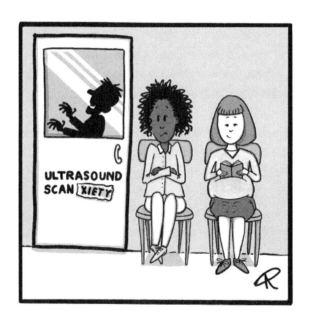

With the right support, it can be a magical experience

We had a rough start to our parenting journey. We experienced difficulty conceiving – three miscarriages within one year, until our healthy daughter was born.

In order for me to share what worked throughout that pregnancy, I need to share my story. Woven throughout are all the many things that helped us along this fourth time, which I am sure were the many reasons why this pregnancy made it to the end and with a healthy baby, and how I survived pregnancy after loss mentally as well.

All my pregnancies were after the age of forty. It took a while to conceive which then happened easily after I had two laparoscopes, initially to do some fertility investigation, and then again to properly remove the endometriosis that was found.

Unfortunately, we lost all three of our babies during that first trimester. We don't know the reasons for our first two miscarriages. We had genetic testing of our third tiny girl and found out it was a random genetic error – nothing we could have done or controlled – the baby was mono-chromosomal: a single X chromosome indicating Turner's syndrome.

As we proceeded to try for a fourth pregnancy, we thought we'd give ourselves more of a chance of a viable pregnancy by trying IVF with PGS (pre-implantation genetic screening) testing to check for normal embryos, thereby reducing the chance of another miscarriage. We visited a fertility specialist to get the ball rolling and as soon as we'd completed all the admin requirements, we started our first IVF cycle.

Alongside this medical treatment, I'd been preparing my body, and mind, for a long time with a variety of complementary medicines, therapies and support, which I'm sure contributed to our goal of having a baby: food sensitivity testing for me and my partner, diet changes, regular acupuncture, Chinese herbs, nutritional supplements, craniosacral therapy, and occasional massage therapy, osteopathy, and several womb and fertility massage treatments – which I eventually trained in! I also did self-fertility massage, castor oil packs, yoni steaming, women's circles, miscarriage workshops, yoga, meditation, decreased stress, a year of doula training, a LOT of mindset work, listened to birth podcasts, and did gratitude journaling. Leigh, my husband, also did all the diet, nutritional supplements, and herbal medicines, too.

On our first cycle of IVF, I gave myself the injections, and alongside all my nutritional supplements and herbs, I took prednisolone and aspirin (a standard protocol to prevent miscarriage). I later started progesterone pessaries. As you can see, we did EVERYTHING!

It looked like we had a lot of follicles growing – each potentially containing an egg – and the uterine lining was nice and thick. Thankfully, due to everything I was doing to support this medical intervention, I had no side effects to the medications, which is unusual. When it was time to have our egg collection, we ended up with only five eggs.

Only three of these eggs were mature. Two of them fertilized. That made two embryos. I know that's not a lot, but we were so fortunate to have them. Not everyone gets this far. In the end, we decided not to do the PGS testing and take our chances, due to time and expense. Then it was a waiting game to see if they'd divide and develop over a few days. We were going to do a 'fresh' transfer where they place the embryo into your uterus straight away, but we discovered we'd missed the ideal window, so these embryos would be frozen after three days of development, and we'd do a frozen transfer (FET) the following month.

As we approached the right time for our FET, an embryo was thawed, and thankfully, survived the thaw. Phew. Would it continue to split and develop so we could transfer? Unfortunately, we were told that it didn't look like this embryo was going anywhere, so would we like to thaw the other embryo? Our last precious embryo. One last chance. We agreed to thaw and hoped for the best. It survived the thaw and looked OK. The transfer was scheduled for the next morning.

I drove to the clinic, ready to become PUPO (pregnant until proven otherwise) that very day. I was met with some surprising news. The second embryo hadn't continued to grow and would be discarded. No options left. However, the embryologist said that the first embryo looked like it might be doing something, but they weren't overly hopeful. The plan was to give it until the next day and see how things unfolded.

I went home and prepared for the worst news in the morning. I thought about that little embryo and hoped it was resilient. Grow, embryo, grow! The next morning, I received the shock of my life when I was told that this embryo had continued to develop into a partial morula. The scientists and doctors were surprised. Although this wasn't the greatest amount of development, it was good enough for me. I went in for my transfer. The procedure was quick and easy.

I spent the next few days at home just nourishing myself and connecting with baby. No work or anything else. I remember this time very fondly. Lots of resting, keeping warm, eating nourishing foods, enjoying acupuncture, music, visualization, and connecting with my baby in any way that I could think of.

We had our two-week wait to find out if it worked. I treated myself as though I was pregnant, hopeful that our resilient baby had implanted and was growing and thriving. The only symptom I remember was being exhausted. And I hoped it was for a good reason! At the end of the two-week wait, I did a home pregnancy test in the morning before going in for my blood test. It was a quick and strong positive! I was somehow not surprised that it was positive. Yet at the same time, I was so shocked that it all worked. I still can't believe it! We had one questionably viable embryo. One cycle. One-shot. And it worked.

I had to trust that our miracle, who'd fought to make it this far, would stick around. Since I'd lost babies at eight, nine and twelve weeks, I was desperate to pass these milestones which I thought would bring me some relief. My mantra was all about surrendering, trusting, and believing. I had my moments, trust me, but mostly, I truly believed we'd end up with a healthy baby at the end.

I did everything I could to reduce stress in my life (mostly!). I continued all my supportive therapies and took my supplements and medications. I commissioned a yogi and naturopath to create a pregnancy after loss yoga series for my online PAL program and used it myself, which was SO helpful. I did Spinning Babies postures/positions/yoga most days. I loved being pregnant.

Although I was anxious at times that this pregnancy wouldn't last, because miscarriages were my only experience of pregnancy, I was also happy and excited. All the way through, I'd pass by a mirror, catch sight of my bump, and be surprised and delighted. Leigh and I would often say to each other: "Can you believe there's a baby in there!"

In the first trimester, my main symptoms were fatigue and sore breasts. I had a little nausea but nothing significant. As long as I had those symptoms during the first part of the pregnancy, that meant I was still pregnant. If you've had a miscarriage, you'll know that usually, those symptoms disappear. So as long as they were there, everything was OK for me. I would check my boobs daily for soreness! Occasionally, I would think the soreness was gone and it would freak me out. You'll know exactly what I mean if you've experienced this.

So, happily, the pregnancy carried on. We agreed to have a scan at seven weeks to give us peace of mind that there was a viable pregnancy. It was a joyful relief to see my tiny little baby with a healthy beating heart. My preference was to have a low intervention pregnancy and birth. So, we organized a home birth, and booked private midwives, a doula, and a birth photographer. We had the dream team!

We held off having any more scans except for the twenty-week anatomy scan. Again, just before the scan, I was nervous we'd find something wrong. But I was again reassured that everything was perfect. We got an amazing profile shot of the baby, and both of us immediately commented how the baby looked just like Leigh! We didn't find out the gender; we wanted it to be a sweet surprise. Initially, we both felt that this was a boy, but towards the end of the pregnancy, I felt it was a girl.

We sailed along through our pregnancy with no complications. As mentioned, we kept it intervention minimal, so I declined most of the usual things offered. Working with independent midwives also meant that there was no unnecessary focus on my age or anything else. The baby and I continued to be perfectly healthy. Our appointments were usually about an hour, giving me all the time needed to discuss anything. This was wonderful for keeping everything stress-free and I highly recommend it, even if you are planning a hospital birth!

Add to this my regular appointments with my doula, which were full of conversation and bodywork, and this all helped me to stay grounded throughout the pregnancy and not float off into space with unrealistic thoughts about what could go wrong.

Around thirty-five weeks we decided to have a babymoon. I was speaking at a conference at the Gold Coast, and we added a few days on to make it a little holiday together. The last chance before the birth! That was a great experience. The conference was amazing – a practitioner business conference where I learnt loads and hung out with all my practice besties as well as meeting many new ones. And I was able to do a talk about miscarriage and pregnancy after loss to my colleagues.

Around 38/39 weeks, my midwife became concerned that I was measuring quite large, so I agreed to have an ultrasound scan to double check. The worst-case scenario was polyhydramnios which meant excessive amniotic fluid, possible complications and interventions for the birth. I freaked out. I had the scan. Turns out, I just make a lot of fluid. It was a high normal, but still within normal limits. The baby was fine. Everything was fine. What a relief. We didn't have to intervene in any way. This was the only 'scare' during the pregnancy, thankfully.

I felt pretty great during the pregnancy. I was so grateful to make it to each milestone and allowed myself to believe, (most of the time), that we were actually going to have a baby. As we approached our estimated due date, people asked if I wanted the baby 'out' ASAP. I said many times that I was feeling fine and happy to go to forty-two weeks if the baby wasn't ready before then. Famous last words!

Our forty-week guess date came and went. That was no problem for me or my midwives. Baby and I were perfectly well. As we approached forty-two weeks, I was curious as to how long this pregnancy would continue. At forty-one weeks plus five days, I remember laying in bed on my side before turning out the light and then heard a pop and a gush, and said to Leigh, "I think my waters just broke!" and jumped out of bed. Getting back into bed with a towel, I wondered when the contractions would start.

After a marathon four and a half days of labor – a big story for another time – our baby was born. She was healthy. And I couldn't believe she was real, that she was ours, and we got to keep her. Such is pregnancy after loss.

As you can see, there were so many things that helped us this time around to maintain our sanity, health, and hope during pregnancy following three losses. If I had to choose one thing that helped the most, it was having a supportive birth team that supported all of our wishes, without judgement, and with continuity of care. Private midwives, a doula, and even a supportive birth photographer sometimes acting as a doula, were the most invaluable.

Pregnancy after loss is tough, and anyone who has experienced this understands the innocence lost, the anxiety and the daily ups and downs. But with the right support, it can be a magical experience.

Grace Miano @thegracemiano

Infertility doesn't end with two pink lines

After years of trying to conceive, I thought the moment we saw two pink lines all our worries and anxiety would slowly fade to the background as those two pink lines grew stronger. Wrong.

Years of trying to conceive, followed by countless monitored and medicated cycles at our fertility clinic, failed IUIs, rounds of IVF and a miscarriage left us permanently scarred. We had 'infertility hangover.'

Pregnancy after infertility and loss is terrifying.Everything, your efforts, your thoughts, your emotions, your finances – everything you've put into creating this life feels like it now lies delicately within your abdomen. I'm a rational person and I knew the data; the stats; the science; the recommendations. I *knew* that my previous actions didn't cause our infertility or our miscarriage. But I still doubted and questioned everything.

Did I drink too much coffee? Did I sleep on my back when I shouldn't have? Should I have gone on that run? Am I eating enough or the right nutrients? Should I paint my nails? Every. Single. Daily. Action. Was. Questioned. And every tingle, cramp or ligament pain was cause for over analysis and panic. Especially early on.

Far from our anxiety disappearing, it seemed to be compounded. We had *so much* at stake. We'd finally created a life. Now we had nine torturous months to wait to meet him and obsess over Every. Little. Thing.

We waited anxiously for every milestone. But after our elation over betas doubling, or graduating from our fertility clinic to our OB, the fear and anxiety would settle right back in. Milestones were like a drug; we couldn't wait for the next 'hit' – but we'd crash back down afterwards.

As the weeks went on, the milestones became more significant, for example, passing week twenty-four – often thought of as the first week outside of the womb that the baby would have a chance of surviving. From then on, the anxiety subsided and we welcomed our perfect baby boy to much elation and celebration at thirty-eight weeks.

We were amazed and in awe when we were able to conceive our second son via spontaneous pregnancy. One would think after having a smooth pregnancy, the anxiety would ease the next time around. Wrong again. Being a spontaneous pregnancy, we had significantly less early pregnancy monitoring. All of a sudden, I was a 'normal' pregnant mother, and my infertility hangover was raging. The reassurances we had during our first pregnancy – multiple beta tests, early ultrasounds, pre-genetic screening – vanished the second time around. And the fear was crippling. But once again, momentary calm ensued following each milestone until we were, once again, able to enjoy the anticipation and excitement. And then we welcomed our second little miracle, again, at thirty-eight weeks.

The infertility hangover made us question whether we should try to have a third. Was that pushing our luck? Who were *we* – an 'infertile' couple – to try to have a THIRD child? There was a time when we didn't even think we could have one. After serious consideration, we set a time limit for trying to conceive. We couldn't face being in that TTC limbo for an unending period as we had for so many years. We were, miraculously, able to conceive spontaneously once more during our timelines. And once again, the fears and anxiety set in. That feeling of 'pushing our luck' – even now at twenty-eight weeks pregnant as I write this – still hangs over my head. The milestones have helped. Feeling her kicks are always reassuring. But it's still a nerve-wracking experience and scary to even write these words down!

Infertility is a long, hard road. It shapes you as a person. It changes your outlook. For better, for worse. And it alters the course you thought your life would take. The experience impacted me so greatly that it created a change in my career. I left my corporate role in brand management to help start myMindBodyBaby Inc., an online community to provide trusted, researched-based fertility lifestyle resources to support fertility and conception.

Research has proven that the right nutrition, movement, and mental well-being can lead to an improved fertility status, higher clinical pregnancy and live birth rates. We partner with fertility clinics and connect online with those struggling to conceive to provide our fertility treatment tailored programs – diet guidance including meal plans, mental health support and motivation, plus fertility-safe fitness and workout videos. Upon the request of fertility clinics, we also have a nutritional, exercise, and mental well-being program for those in the first trimester after fertility treatment to help ease early pregnancy anxiety.

Because infertility doesn't end with two pink lines.

Lyndsey Clabby @mymindbodybaby

A case of the guilts

The first time I found out I was pregnant, I was overjoyed. My dream to be a parent was coming true. After hearing the heartbeat of our baby on the eight-week scan, we bought a twin pack of baby suits to mark the occasion, blissfully unaware that anything could go wrong and clueless about the challenges ahead of us.

Fast forward and I'm now writing this at thirty weeks, the furthest I've got in any of my pregnancies. After four miscarriages, I should be overjoyed, but when I discovered I was pregnant again, I was terrified. I still can't forget we'd been here before and all those times ended badly. I want to be excited, and I truly am, but I can't shake this worry that something bad will happen. And I feel guilty for having those thoughts.

I thought that my battle was staying pregnant, but it hasn't stopped there. I've had many complications along the way which only amplified the fear and worry. But I keep telling myself I haven't come this far to give up now. But it's not easy being pregnant after loss. And it's ok to admit that. It's also very understandable given the circumstances. It doesn't make me ungrateful. It's just the trauma from the recurrent loss that still haunts me.

With each passing milestone, I've hoped a switch would be flicked and I could finally relax; that when I got to twelve weeks it would all be fine (the furthest I'd ever got in a pregnancy was eleven weeks). Or I'd get to twenty weeks (halfway) or twenty-four weeks (viability) or twenty-eight weeks (third trimester), and I'd feel as overjoyed as I did in that first pregnancy. That didn't happen this time, and I'm not sure it will.

It's only recently that I've been able to buy things for the baby. I still feel so anxious setting up the nursery, thinking my baby might not get to spend any time there and that I'll come home from the hospital empty-handed to a house surrounded by baby things. I'm on the home stretch of this pregnancy now, but I know I won't be able to relax until my baby is safely in my arms. Although some have told me that its once baby arrives, that the worry really starts!

It's so important not to beat ourselves up if our experience of pregnancy after loss isn't all rosy. There's no pressure. Allow yourself to feel how you need to feel, because acknowledging those emotions is the first step in dealing with them. And when you can, allow yourself a break from those negative feelings and make space for some positive ones too – the hope, excitement and happiness. It's possible to feel fear and hope, worry and excitement, anxiety and happiness. You don't have to choose. You do you.

Nora @thislimboland

Excitement was replaced with fear

Pregnancy after infertility was something I wasn't sure I'd ever experience. When we found out in 2017 that we had a .02% chance of having genetic children, our world crashed around us. So, the idea that I'd ever fall pregnant and experience this milestone, seemed out of reach. That was until we were introduced to embryo donation adoption (EDA). There are about 1,000,000 frozen embryos in the United States alone from couples who went through IVF and are storing their remaining embryos. When a couple has completed their family, they have the option to donate their remaining embryos to a family, who was like us, were unable to have genetic children. When we heard this option, we knew right away that this was the right option. We finally felt like we were on the path to becoming parents and the idea of carrying a baby seemed more real.

When we finally transferred our embryo from our donor's batch and got pregnant, what should have been excitement was replaced with absolute fear. Every step became harder and harder. And I told myself that after the next beta, I'd feel better, or once I saw a heartbeat, I'd be able to breathe, or once I make it to another week, I'd be okay. Desperation built up at each milestone and I never felt confident. I was waiting for my body to fail me.

The waiting between appointments and ultrasounds was torture. I'd constantly be worried they wouldn't be able to find a heartbeat and we'd lose the baby. The constant fear made pregnancy almost unbearable. I was always holding my breath until I heard the heartbeat or watched the baby do flips on the ultrasound. And when I heard or saw what I needed for reassurance, that fear vanished only to return when the appointment was over. And then the cycle began again, holding my breath until the next appointment.

I missed out on those many amazing moments that someone who doesn't have infertility or loss experiences, such as weekly 'bump' photos. I didn't get round to taking any until I was twenty-six weeks pregnant. In fact, I didn't really take many pictures at all while pregnant. My sister wanted to organise a baby shower when I was twelve weeks gone, and I couldn't even wrap my head around it. I didn't want to celebrate our baby until I was at least thirty weeks in case something bad happened. Decorating and preparing the nursery was also something I waited to do past thirty weeks. My recurrent thoughts were, *what if we never bring our baby home?*

Infertility and loss robs you of all those beautiful moments that you waited so long for. It takes any bit of excitement and replaces it with fear. You hold your breath the entire time to protect your heart. Then if something happens, you tell yourself, "I knew it would end like this." And you torment yourself the entire pregnancy until you're holding your baby in your arms. Even then, you aren't crying tears of joy; you're crying because you're able to breathe a sigh of relief because your baby made it. And so did you.

Kate Knapton @jojiiandco

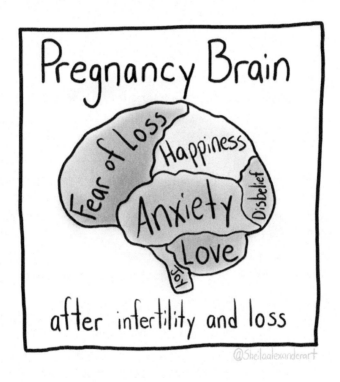

Why me? Why not her?

Why me? Why not her? How ironic it is that while going through infertility, I often asked myself this. Why did this happen to me and not her? And yet, when I became pregnant, the same questions plagued me, just in a different context. Why did I get pregnant, and she didn't?

When I got the call from the clinic that my IVF transfer was a success, I was elated and beyond grateful. For four years, I'd gotten so used to disappointment and hearing the word "No," that this newfound "Yes," I yearned for, for so long, seemed hard to believe. I was truly in disbelief. Relief swept over me. And so did guilt. I couldn't help but think of those still struggling. Why me? Why not her?

I decided to focus on gratitude. With gratitude came compassion and empathy for those still in the wait. It was deeply important to me to acknowledge others on their journeys. I remember several friends, telling me not to worry about others and to focus on my pregnancy, but my heart felt otherwise. I knew I could still feel joy while also making others feel 'seen'. So, my behavior was intentional in big and small ways. Waiting to publicly share my pregnancy until I was seven months pregnant allowed me time to process all of the emotions that come with pregnancy after infertility. I also made a point to check in personally with women whose journeys were still underway. I hadn't forgotten about them just because I'd become pregnant. I also went through an odd phase of feeling out of place. When infertility becomes a huge part of your identity, especially on social media, you suddenly find yourself wondering: 'What do I talk about now?'

The important thing is to embrace each new season as it comes, being authentic to who you are and what your heart feels. We live in a very self-centred society, and we are encouraged to focus on our own happiness and success. I believe in celebrating our joys. We should never feel we have to hide our happiness. But in addition to that, if you also choose to serve others, see the value in honoring others' feelings. Do it! I have no regrets in how I navigated pregnancy after infertility, and am so grateful for all the journeys I've been able to be a part of as a result.

Christina Oberon @xtina.o__

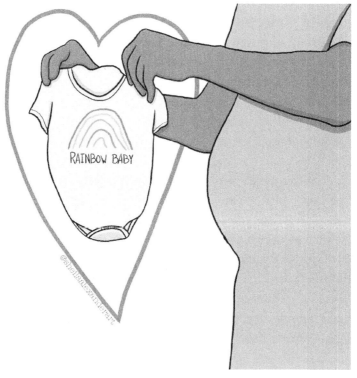

A rainbow baby's first outfit

We are allowed to feel more than one emotion at a time

Pregnancy after the loss of a baby is truly a unique experience. But you have to live through it to really understand. I was constantly feeling a whirlwind of emotions which made it difficult to enjoy my pregnancy.

They say ignorance is bliss and I miss that naivety new mothers have. But that horse had long bolted because I knew all the things that could go wrong during a pregnancy. Because I'd lived it. That was my reality.

As weeks turned into months, pregnancy with my rainbow baby felt like constantly holding my breath. I tried my hardest to enjoy all the moments, to take all the photos, to do all the things I didn't get to with her brother, Damani. Every appointment, I held my breath until they found her heartbeat. All I could do was pray this baby came home with us, alive.

I took a social media absence as everything was too overwhelming. I decided to give myself some grace and take care of my mental health. At times, I felt guilty I was leaving my little boy, Damani behind, but he was very much present in our lives.

As we embraced being a family of four, he was included in the maternity photo shoot and the baby shower; two events we didn't get to have with him.

When Mila was born, we were thankful she didn't require an NICU stay and was absolutely perfect. She wore Damani's socks in the hospital, and when she came home, she also wore his baby clothes. It was heart-breaking, though, that she was wearing hand-me-downs that were never worn by him.

I want people to know that motherhood looks different to the mom or dad parenting after the death of their baby. Mila isn't a replacement for Damani and we're fully aware of the missing member of our family. Although our hearts are incredibly full, there'll always be space for him. Human beings are complex and we're allowed to feel more than one emotion at a time. While we're truly grateful for our sweet little girl, we're also saddened that Damani is dead and his sister will never get to make memories with him. Not everyone will understand that. Some will say, "Be grateful you have a child". But two opposing emotions can still be relevant and we won't invalidate Damani's life.

To those pregnant after the death of their baby, be kind to yourself; take time to bond and savour every moment; capture all those memories. We know how life can change in an instant. How pictures can be all you have left. Find a supportive doctor and healthcare team, reach out to people who understand and have been there. And remember, you're not alone.

Crystal-Gayle @4Damani

Pregnancy after loss - anxiety and doubts

Instagram post October 27th 2021

For real though - pregnancy after loss can be crippled with anxiety, fears, doubts, and more. And for me, not only did we have four losses after our first son, but I wasn't able to carry our second, and I was explicitly told by multiple doctors that I would never carry another pregnancy...

So as I hold this miracle in my belly:

I am both in awe and scared.
I am grateful and terrified.
I am hopeful and weary.
I am happy and nervous.
I am accepting and fighting denial.
I am excited and anxious.
I want time to go faster and time to slow down.
I want to just have him in my arms, but I want to enjoy the pregnancy.

And so much more...

Pregnancy after loss is a series of contradictions, constantly circling around my mind, and fighting each other for attention and acknowledgement. So, each day, I make a conscious effort to try to accept the good. To believe that this is good and only good. That my body is capable of carrying this child, and my body IS carrying this child now!

I have this thought that when we finally bring him into the world, and I hear him cry - I'll think, OMG, I did it! My body really did it. And I keep holding onto that moment of hope and happiness, and I happily cry thinking about the moment we first see him, and hear him cry. I cannot wait. About 75 days baby boy. 75 days to you.

Instagram post 12 Dec 2021

Tomorrow I'll be 36 weeks pregnant, and I cannot believe we only have about 4 weeks until baby boy joins our family! And I am beyond grateful and blessed that our family will be complete with our three beautiful boys.

But having a child, being pregnant, having multiple children - it doesn't erase the losses. It doesn't erase infertility. It doesn't erase the trauma. And I would never expect a child to heal me, but it can still be harder than expected.

I learned this the hard way with Dylan - I naively thought that when we finally had him, I would be magically healed. I wouldn't have the residual feelings from our four losses and many years of infertility. I don't know why I thought that – I didn't expect him to heal me himself, I would never put that burden on him. But I just expected to be able to move on, without the past creeping in.

But I was wrong. Even though I didn't give birth to Dylan myself, the feelings I had after he was born were confusing. I was so incredibly grateful, so relieved, so joyful... but I was also anxious, terrified, and more. I started having the worst nightmares, that felt VERY real, that something terrible was happening to our boys. I would wake up unsure what happened for real and not. I couldn't sleep well. I worried constantly. And I felt like I couldn't give enough of myself to anyone. I felt like a horrible mother.

So I got help. I starting talking with a therapist – I immediately released more tears and feelings that I didn't even realize still existed in me.

This time I'm feeling more prepared. I've already been doing the work to acknowledge and move through feelings and pain and trauma, and I'm hopeful that if those PPA feelings or more do resurface, I'll have more tools at my disposable to work through them again.

Alex Kornswiet @ourbeautifulsurprise

What I wish I'd known

Being pregnant after infertility and/or loss is a real conundrum. You're so achingly desperate to see two positive lines, but at the same time, so very scared that there'll actually be two lines. You'd think two opposing emotions couldn't sit side by side, but they can, and frequently do. It's easy to allow anxiety to be the main player here and nobody would blame you. After all, you've been through so much already that even buying a pregnancy test creates mixed emotions. "I don't know why I'm bothering to buy it; it'll be negative. But what if it isn't?" And "Do I want to buy the one that unkindly tells me I'm not pregnant? But what if I am and it tells me: 'Pregnant: 2-3 weeks?'" Just this one small but important part of finally being pregnant is already so hard.

When I was finally expecting after six years of unexplained in-fertility and early pregnancy loss, there weren't people sharing their stories on social media or talking openly about navigating these nine months. I should have been floating on cloud nine with a permanent smile on my face, but, instead, I felt as if I was in a black hole, peeking out only when it felt safe.

To be honest, the dreaded two-week wait was the easiest part. I was in ignorant bliss – PUPO (pregnant until proven otherwise), and that was good enough for me. Then when the hCG level came back really high, my anxiety soon kicked in. The last time I was pregnant, I lost our baby, so there was no guarantee I wouldn't lose this one. Of course, this pregnancy was a different egg and sperm, so a new embryo, and also my womb lining wasn't the same as before because it never is exactly the same as a previous pregnancy, and I was on more medication after new tests.

We chose to tell our families and friends straight away. Some knew we'd had fertility treatment, and then an early pregnancy loss only a few months previously. And to be honest, the support even months later from those who hadn't had the "We're pregnant!" news when we did tell them about our miscarriage, was almost non-existent. This time, I wanted more support and empathy if the worst happened. But it's important to do what's right for you. Many women don't say anything until they are sixteen or twenty weeks for various reasons. And that's OK.

Thankfully, I got past the scary six-week mark, but when I shared my concerns that I might lose this baby at some point, many didn't understand: "It won't happen again, that was a one-off," "Be happy you're pregnant," "Stop worrying," or "Just relax". And we all know how upsetting it is when your feelings aren't validated. By empathising, the person feels heard, acknowledged, and understood. It doesn't take much to listen rather than attempt to fix someone.

There was a plus side to my tumultuous emotions. I should've stopped the Clexane (a blood-thinning injection) at twelve weeks, but I had a gut feeling it wasn't a good idea. There was no medical necessity to remain on it, but at my antenatal appointment with the Consultant, I insisted. I even changed Consultants because this first one wouldn't agree. Going through infertility and pregnancy loss taught me to advocate for myself and my baby, and I wasn't leaving that appointment until they accepted my decision. I continued with the injections until I was thirty-four weeks.

I also saw the Consultant regularly throughout my pregnancy because I was forty-six, and at each appointment, she did an ultrasound scan. It might sound strange, but I loved having so many scans. The first one at six weeks was naturally stressful – there's a reason it's called *scanxiety*! But as my pregnancy progressed and everything went well, I looked forward to them, and it was reassuring for myself and my partner to see our baby growing.

However, I wasn't permanently attached to an ultrasound machine, so between appointments, the usual negative thoughts prevailed. For example, I didn't have early morning sickness or cravings like many pregnant women. Some would say I was lucky, but that nagging voice in my head said, "You can't really be pregnant, then." I'd even panic about going to the toilet in case I saw blood. That was one of my biggest worries, and I know I'm not alone. I'd gingerly pull down my knickers and look at anything else in the bathroom rather than 'down there.' After I wiped, through squinted eyes, I'd glance at the scrunched-up paper. No red streak. And breathe. I was still pregnant.

I now know these emotions aren't unusual, but I wish there'd been stories I could've read where others expressed the same emotions. It would have helped me feel normal and maybe I could've enjoyed my one and only pregnancy a little more. Don't get me wrong, I loved being pregnant, but for so long I hadn't had much to celebrate, so, looking back, I spent the entire nine months in shock. Here are some things that I think would've helped me:

- had counselling/therapy to manage my anxiety, and the PTSD I didn't know I had until after giving birth.
- took more bump photos – I'm so glad we did a photo shoot a couple of weeks before I gave birth, but I wish we'd done more throughout the pregnancy.
- kept a journal – if the worst happened, I would've had something to connect me to that time. And as there was a happy ending, it would be part of my and my daughter's story.
- read pregnancy books – though, this could've been because I used to be a midwife and didn't think I needed to.
- brought all the Mother and Baby magazines – just because I could!
- given myself permission to buy some baby clothes whilst pregnant rather than only window shopping.
- knitted some newborn jumpers – yes, I can knit, and I'm cross with myself that I didn't. Thankfully my Mum did.
- had a baby shower/celebration.
- looked for a support group specifically for women who were finally pregnant, though I'm not sure there was any back then.

Despite everything, I had an amazing pregnancy with many memorable moments, connecting with my baby and experiencing the incredible changes my body went through. Fast forward, and I now have a wonderful daughter.

Sheila Lamb @fertilitybooks

The anxiety of not knowing

Alyssa shares her story below. She's still trying to take her baby home. Stories of hope are so important when you are finally pregnant, but the sad reality is, it doesn't always work out how we want. If you'd rather not read Alyssa's story, she understands, but even if you don't, please hold space for Alyssa, her husband and her babies. Thank you.

My husband and I started trying to conceive a little over two years ago. We were hopeful, excited, and naive. After many months of trying, multiple losses, and the rupture of my Fallopian Tube, we got nervous. I booked an appointment with my OB to discuss seeing an RE. Within a few weeks, I was sitting in my new RE's office listening to him say: "You have two uteri (uteruses) and one tube. You won't be able to get pregnant naturally. Let's talk about IVF!"

I'd previously had surgery on my tube due to an ectopic pregnancy, but the doctor had told us that the tube remained open. However, my RE noted that in the minute by minute surgery report, it specifically stated that the tube was closed. Doctors in the past had missed this. We were naturally upset that this mistake was made, but we were eager to move forward with IVF.

I was born with two uteri and the uterus attached to the working tube wasn't accessible. We didn't ask many questions, just signed on the dotted line, and thanked our RE. To be honest, we didn't even grieve the loss of being able to conceive naturally. We were traumatized by our losses, but we still had hope. IVF and loss hadn't defined us. Not yet at least.

We started IVF right away and had amazing results. In October of 2019, we transferred a perfect little boy embryo. The two-week wait, the time between the embryo transfer and pregnancy blood draw, is one of the hardest. Especially after a loss. I was constantly taking pregnancy tests to ensure the line got darker, which reveals the hCG is rising, and the baby is growing. I remember going to the store at 2 a.m. to buy a new test, just so I could confirm I was still pregnant. I spent hundreds of dollars on tests, thousands of minutes waiting, and countless anxiety-induced tears.

We ended up having a few hCG blood draws taken because the numbers weren't rising the way they should have. The anxiety surrounding this was hard to cope with. So much goes into an IVF transfer. The embryo, the shots, the waiting. It's tough to know that you're pregnant, but not know if your baby is growing. In the end, we were able to confirm the pregnancy at week six via ultrasound. He was perfect!

Pregnancy after loss is crippling. It's truly all-consuming. You're closely tracking each milestone and just praying that your baby is going to be okay, that this time will be different. Because I had an ectopic, I spent weeks four to six worried the baby might have implanted again somewhere outside of my uterus. Then, once we had a placement scan to confirm the baby had implanted correctly, I worried I'd miscarry again. Miscarriages without explanations are hard because you don't know how to prevent it from happening again. You're always waiting for the bad news, and when bad news is all you know, it's hard to get excited.

Our sweet little boy made it to nine weeks and we graduated from our RE clinic and onto our OB. The pregnancy was hard from the beginning. I was high risk and seen almost weekly. We also got uncertain first and second-trimester results, which sent me spiraling. I was unable to feel connected to this baby. And the more he grew, the more uncertain I became, having trouble eating, sleeping, and socializing with pregnant friends, especially those who'd never experienced loss before. I refused to buy anything for our baby, and despite my growing tummy, my partner and I, couldn't even talk about names. We were terrified.

Our little boy ended up needing an amnio, and by week eighteen, we realized something serious was going on. These were the hardest weeks of my life. Praying that he was okay but knowing he probably wasn't. By week twenty-two a Whole Exome Gene Sequencing test confirmed our worst nightmare – we'd lose our son, Cole, to a rare genetic defect.

The following Saturday, I ended up in the delivery emergency room diagnosed with Adjustment Disorder and heavily medicated. On Friday, March 20th, 2020, one week into the pandemic, we lost our son at twenty-three weeks. It was a multiple day process that I remember like yesterday. We had about an hour with Cole before we had to say goodbye. It will forever remain the most heartbreakingly beautiful moment of my life. The weeks following the loss are still a blur. I could barely get out of bed. It's hard to navigate how to deal with the postpartum period without your baby, while also grieving his loss and being stuck at home during a pandemic. It wasn't until my first postpartum menstrual period came that I felt myself again. I started to regain hope.

We did PGD testing for the single gene defect on the remaining eleven embryos and were left with seven healthy embryos. Hope. We had SO much hope. That's what kept us going. Losing our baby was hard. It was probably the hardest thing we will ever have to go through as a couple. I just remember thinking, I am SO grateful for science and technology. Without it, we wouldn't have been able to identify Cole's defect. We wouldn't have been able to test our remaining embryos to ensure we didn't suffer a loss like that again. And we wouldn't be where we are today, one step closer to a healthy pregnancy and baby.

On June 16th, 2020, just three months postpartum, we transferred another embryo. Another boy. We had so much hope during the TWW. I saw rainbows EVERYWHERE. We knew this was it. I could feel it in my heart. Until suddenly, I got the call. It was negative. We cried. We felt defeated. But I wasn't ready to stop.

We continued with four more transfers. All negative. Every two-week wait was harder than the last. We kept losing embryos and no one could give us any answers.

Until July 2021! It was our sixth transfer and my fourth time seeing those two pink lines. It worked! We were pregnant again. I remember being in shock. My husband didn't believe it was real. I peed on twenty-six pregnancy tests during the wait for the blood draw. It was the longest wait of my life. I was bleeding and absolutely terrified. But my HCG looked good, and my doctor told me to hang on a little longer in hope that we'd soon see our wiggly little baby on the ultrasound screen.

I was so anxious after so much loss that I asked the doctor to see me at five weeks and five days for a scan. It was very early, but I couldn't wait any longer. I wasn't sleeping and I knew the stress wasn't good for the baby. But that's something many women struggle with while pregnant after a loss. They are told to stay calm, that this time is better, that the baby will be okay, that stress isn't good for the baby. But how do you not feel stressed when things have gone wrong in the past?

After my scan, my doctor found the pregnancy quickly, but all that was there was an empty sac. "It's still early. Let's give it a few more days. Come back on Monday and we'll assess." I, again, was asked to go home and wait to see if my baby was okay.

My baby wasn't okay. It was a blighted ovum. It looked like our little girl tried to split into two sacs; something went wrong and she stopped growing. Another loss for us. I now wondered how my fifth pregnancy would be? After an ectopic, nine-week miscarriage, twenty-three-week late loss, and seven-week blighted ovum, how will I ever be able to survive the anxiety that comes with pregnancy after loss?

We haven't lost hope, but I am a changed woman because of these experiences. These losses have defined my well-being, my life.

Alyssa @healthyivf

What worked for us

As my wife and I left our footloose and fancy-free young adult life, we focused on what many refer to as 'the next step.' It was time to start a family. How hard could that be?

Let's face it, many people spend years trying to avoid getting pregnant, so we thought this would be a cinch, right? Well, not so much. My wife and I experienced multiple losses before the birth of our first child. At the time, we were unaware of how common it is for pregnancies to be lost. But if it happens so often, why are we all so ill-prepared?

There's no way to effectively ready yourself for loss. Nobody boards an airplane fully prepared for the jet to fall out of the sky. In the back of your mind, you know that the possibility is there, but you're all but certain it won't happen to you. However, in every decision we make lies the acceptance of the risks.

As a husband, I wanted to be sure that I was the ultimate support system for my wife through every one of our pregnancies. She had more than her fair share of things to worry about physically, let alone the fear of recurring pregnancy loss. Because of this, common occurrences such as spotting or cramping became terrifying. This made every milestone or appointment an exercise in holding our breath where we pleaded with the universe to hear a pounding heartbeat on the ultrasound. Having been to appointments where the outcome ended both happily as well as tragically, it became clear, nothing prepares you for either result. The symphony of elation that overcomes you when you hear the tha-thump, tha-thump of your little one's tiny, healthy heart for the first time or the sound of the planet grinding to a halt when the only feedback is silence; it's beyond overwhelming.

What was important was sharing the incredible news of our unborn child's well-being with loved ones who truly delighted in our excitement. There's nothing worse than having someone react as though they're indifferent. When the news was bad, my wife and I trudged through the misery and darkness together. It was no easy task picking one another up, but it was critical to give each other the time and support to move forward.

It's difficult to know what to recommend to anyone embarking on this journey. When you're at a place in your life when you want something so badly, it's hard to separate emotion from reason. I distinctly remember telling Kim during our first pregnancy, "See, Google says spotting is totally normal." Thirty-six hours later, we were in the ER suffering a crushing loss.

The only thing that saved us was being honest with ourselves and one another. When attempting to climb Mt. Everest, you accept that much can go wrong. Be that as it may, that mountain peak is nothing short of majestic. So, although the road was long and painful, we vowed to stick to that journey together, no matter how it ended. That's what saw us through.

Mark @bombprooffamily

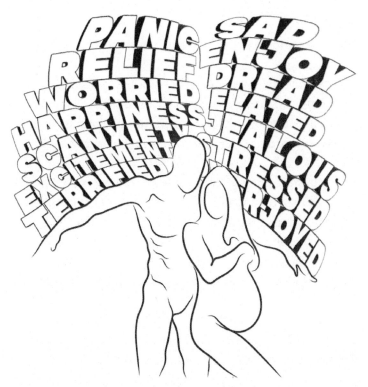

Men and pregnancy after infertility and loss

I found myself moving the goalposts for happiness

"Congratulations! You must be over the moon!"

Finally pregnant after several unsuccessful rounds of fertility treatment, we fully expected to be just that. However, failure and disappointment had taken their toll, and instead, we found ourselves gearing up for the next inevitable knock-back.

From the beginning of my pregnancy, I found myself moving the goalposts for happiness, convinced that I could only enjoy being pregnant after we'd crossed the hurdles ahead of us.
"Once I hear the heartbeat, I'll relax."
"Once I reach twelve weeks I'll stop worrying so much."
"Once I reach the next scan, we can start to believe."

I also insisted that the people around us adopted this cautious approach to our happy news.
"We're expecting a baby! But don't get too excited, it's still early days."

I remember sharing a scan photo at work to a chorus of happy squeals and congratulations but struggled to join in and quickly turned down the suggestion of a baby shower.

It's hard to say exactly when I did enjoy being pregnant. However, I'm so thankful that I did and would encourage anyone feeling similar anxieties to do the same. Having bubble baths staring down at my belly, lazy lie-ins feeling her little kicks and simply walking down the road – being pregnant – finally having my turn at being a Mum. These are just some of the hazy happy memories which I'll always cherish from those early days.

After our daughter was born, we shared our experience of an anxious pregnancy through illustrations on our Instagram page. Amongst the flood of comments from fellow fertility warriors were many heartfelt words of wisdom. If we ever have the privilege of falling pregnant again, I'll follow one of my favourite gems of advice: 'Protecting your heart every step of the way will not stop the pain should the worst happen, so why not choose to lean into your fears, and feel all of the joy of each moment."

I know it's easier said than done but being pregnant is such a special time, don't miss it.

Laura @fertilit_arty

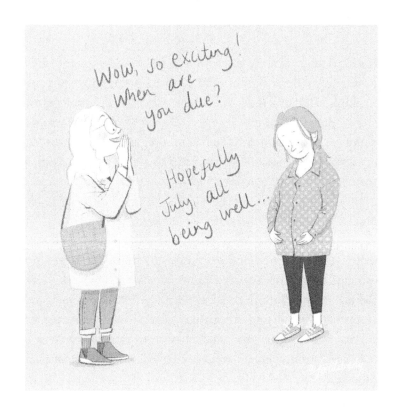

This maternity shoot was something I had to do

From IG post October 26th 2021

One year ago, I got these photos back. I dreamed about this moment, about taking these photos. But I was fearful, I was anxious every day. If I didn't feel her enough, if my boobs stopped hurting, if they hurt too much, if I felt pain or if I didn't, if I was tired or if I wasn't. It didn't matter. I was scared.

But this photo, this maternity shoot was something I had to do, I had to remember my body working for me. I wanted to look back and remember the good, the happy moments in my pregnancy. I wanted to celebrate it, how far we had come, how fast it had gone by, and how, not matter what happened, in that moment I was happy.

I can't believe it's been a year. It feels like a lifetime ago that we took these. And yet, I look at this photo and smile. I remember freezing my butt off, I remember the twins laughing at me because I took my clothes off in the middle of a field (surrounded by houses), I remember thinking that one day I will get to show her these photos and I'm sure she will think it's gross too.

But I also look at this photo and feel a little sad, exhausted because of what it took to get there. Anxious about the thought of trying for that last embryo because of all the steps I know I need to take first, knowing that it might not even result in a pregnancy, like this one.

So here we are, weeks away from her first birthday, staring at what seems like an eternity ago and yet not able to erase any of the feelings that took over my body that day, and most days leading up to it.

Erin Bulcao @mybeautifulblunder

Seven ways to reduce rainbow pregnancy anxiety

Reading other people's stories is really supportive and helps to validate our emotions. But I thought it may also help to read some advice from a therapist who's experienced in pregnancy after infertility and loss.

Conceiving again after a pregnancy loss may seem like a roller-coaster of emotions. Joy and relief may be mixed with anxiety and fear. Many of my clients also share their sense of being on edge next time around; hyper-alert for any signs or symptoms of the pregnancy failing. Pregnancy should be a happy time and now the magic is diluted with worry.

Here are my seven research-backed ways to reduce rainbow pregnancy anxiety. I hope they'll help you.

1. **Support**

Good support makes a huge difference. Build your team. Talk to your partner, family, and friends about what you're feeling. Remember this is a new and different pregnancy. You are continuing your family-building. Some women choose to share their rainbow pregnancy news straight away to feel more connected and savour every moment of being pregnant. Others stay with the three-month announcement when they feel safer. It's an individual choice.

2. **Daily Habits**
Routines are reassuring. When you're eating well, getting outdoors for some exercise, and having enough sleep, you are doing your best for your baby.

3. **Exercise**
Our bodies are designed for movement and our brain wakes up and works better afterwards. Walking outdoors gives you a special benefit which neuroscientists call 'optical flow' as the scenery appears to move past you. This relaxes your gaze and calms your mind. And it's far healthier than staring at a screen.

4. **Affirmations**
If anxiety kicks in and feelings spiral into negative loops, affirmations are a quick way to ground you. These are positive statements to help you overcome negative thoughts. When you have these phrases ready, you can repeat them as often as you need to calm and focus your mind. Useful affirmations may sound like: "This is a healthy pregnancy, a healthy baby", "I deserve to be pregnant", "I am worthy" and "My body is nurturing my baby".

5. **Breathe**
Did you know that breathing changes your thinking? Let me share how the 'Physiological Sigh' works. When you've been crying and go through the 'honking like a goose' stage,

that breathing pattern is two short, sharp inhalations, followed immediately by a long exhalation. I call it 'sniff, sniff, blow'. It feels incredibly good to do. Try it for yourself. Neuroscience studies show this breathing stimulates your diaphragm's phrenic nerve to instantly send a calming message to your brain. Maybe that's why we often feel better after a good cry!

6. **Mindfulness Meditation**
Mindfulness practice is associated with reduced anxiety, improved mood, and better-coping skills in times of uncertainty. It helps you feel more in control of what you can control in your life. And it helps improve things like wellbeing and sleep, contributing to a healthy pregnancy. "I feel more anxious when I try to meditate" is something I hear a lot. An easy way to get into a meditative mindset is doing repetitive movement! Walking, dancing, and knitting train your brain and ease your emotions. Practice makes perfect and there's loads of help to get you started. Guided meditations are a good option on apps or YouTube. They vary in length from ten minutes to over an hour. Thirty minutes is usually enough. Find a few you can enjoy as part of your self-care routine.

7. **Hypnotherapy**
Imagine hitting the 'pause' button in your mind for a while. A skilled therapist tailors your session for your exact needs and can help you with your own mindfulness practice. Hypnotherapy allows you to pause your mind and reset your emotions.

Helena Tubridy @helenatubridy

I couldn't bring myself to click 'buy'

After years of trying to conceive, one miscarriage and one round of IVF, the impossible happened, and we became pregnant. As soon as I saw the positive lines on the pregnancy test, it all felt a bit like a dream. I was so prepared for the IVF not to work, that I hadn't considered how it would feel if it did work. I was happy and excited, running downstairs to shout the news at my husband, but we weren't quite sure how to process the news.

We followed the instructions from our fertility clinic and booked in for the relevant blood tests and scans at six weeks and eight weeks. I was incredibly nervous before every appointment because it felt like our dreamy bubble could be popped at any time. I constantly checked my knickers terrified I'd see blood again, and every day I googled every last symptom, literally anything my body did and felt, in case it meant something bad. After seeing the heartbeat at the scans and then being told after the eight-week scan that we no longer needed to go to the clinic, we felt a little scared. The clinic had looked after us for months and now we were officially pregnant and transferred to the NHS system like a 'normal' couple.

The midwife gave us our purple folder and booked us in for

the twelve-week scan which fell the day after Mother's Day. I hoped that was a good omen? The NHS wasn't geared up for IVF though. I regularly had to explain the irrelevance of when my last period started as I could give them an exact due date. On more than one occasion, I was told: "Well, we have to measure the baby to check," which they did and promptly confirmed I had the right due date.

I was so relieved to see our baby again at the twelve-week scan. This time, our longed-for baby actually resembled one as opposed to the blob we'd seen in previous scans. We watched with fascination as the little life we created did somersaults in my tummy, and happily walked away with our little framed scan image. It still didn't feel real, but now we'd have to start telling people.

After years of being tortured by Facebook pregnancy announcements, we didn't want to share the news on there. Instead, we told a few people discreetly. I found it difficult to accept their enthusiasm or congratulations because, without a bump, I felt a bit like a fraud. It still didn't feel real. I was particularly careful with friends who I knew were struggling with their own infertility issues. I knew all too well how they'd be feeling when I told them our happy news.

For the rest of my pregnancy, I watched in complete amazement as my body underwent huge changes, and people started to see that I was pregnant and talk to me about it. I loved feeling my baby move around but I didn't dare buy any baby stuff yet though. I couldn't bring myself to actually click 'buy' until I was thirty-three weeks pregnant. If anyone gave us an early gift, I kept it wrapped up and hidden away. I was even worried I'd be tempting fate by setting up the nursery; but once we had, the door remained firmly closed.

It wasn't that I didn't enjoy being pregnant; I loved every second of it. I suppose after desperately wanting a child for so long, nothing felt guaranteed, and until my baby was safely in my arms, all of this would continue to be a wonderful dream.

After a complicated birth, thanks to me being induced and it not going to plan, I ended up being wheeled down to the theatre for an emergency caesarean. In under ten minutes, my baby boy was pulled from my tummy. Weirdly, I didn't feel any pain, but I could feel the surgeon rummaging around and then with one big tug, there was that enormous release of my baby being pulled out. I heard a muted little cry and my heart felt like it was going to burst with relief. They quickly checked our baby over, wrapped him up, and my husband brought him over for me to hold. I gazed down at the most beautiful baby in the whole world. He looked up at me and I said, "Hello my love, I've been waiting for you".

"Congratulations Mummy," the midwife said with a huge smile. Gosh, it was all very real then.

Lianne Baker

My overwhelming emotion was anxiety

I was in my thirties when I decided to have a baby on my own. I'd spent the last ten years presuming I'd bump into someone unexpectedly – perhaps, at the supermarket, where our eyes would lock over our shopping baskets, or I'd walk into a meeting at work and there'd be a handsome new employee sat across the desk. I soon came to realise I'd have to put more effort in to make romance happen, yet speed dating, blind dates and internet dating yielded the same poor results. So, at the age of thirty-four, after much research, I made an appointment with my local fertility clinic.

The doctor said three Intra-Uterine Inseminations (IUIs) would give me a good chance of a pregnancy and I began the treatment fully expecting it to take all three tries. So, I was ecstatic to see two pink lines appear on my pregnancy test after my first IUI cycle.

I had three blissful weeks of cradling my belly, talking to my little blob, and imagining our future together. Yet my world was about to come crashing down when at my seven-week scan, I heard those heart-breaking words: "I'm sorry there's no heartbeat". I was devastated.

Three months later, I tried again, and both times, I saw those two pink lines at the same time as the pink lines appeared in my underwear – 'chemical pregnancies' they call them. The pain was real even though the doctor told me they didn't count.

I tried again, desperate to experience that same joy I felt that first time. After another two negative cycles, I was pregnant again. My anxiety was through the roof, but the joy I'd been chasing was weighed down by fear. My stomach was in knots, every twinge feeling like terror. One moment, I was convinced the pains were anxiety and the next certain they were signs my baby was dying. I could barely concentrate on anything other than whether my baby was still alive. I was a zombie at work just trying to get through the day.

At six and a half weeks, I had some bleeding when I went to the toilet. I was at the garden centre with friends and went to the loo. Soon after, they followed me in wondering if I was OK, trying to calm me down with stories about their bleeding through pregnancy, but I knew this was different. The out of hours GP referred me to the Emergency Department who confirmed I was no longer pregnant.

I went on to have another two losses. With the next, I saw a glorious seven-week embryo wriggling around on the screen only for their heart to stop at my nine-week scan. After that, I had another six-week loss.

It all took its toll on me and I had a break from trying to conceive and concentrated on my own well-being for a while. Then I went into my fourteenth IUI, knowing a fifteenth would be my last.

I tested at twelve days post ovulation and saw those two pink lines appear again.

It's a weird mix of contradictory emotions when you see that positive pregnancy test after multiple losses. There's still joy, but it comes with fear, sadness, confusion, guilt, and anger. Fear that I'd lose this baby too; sadness at remembering my other babies that never made it into my arms; guilt that I wasn't feeling happier. And anger that pregnancy loss had stolen my ability to feel unbridled excitement like most people.

It was also isolating going through the pregnancy on my own. I was lucky to have lots of supportive friends and family, but this baby was mine alone and no one else had the same connection to it as I did. If anything happened, I'd be going to bed on my own and waking alone without anyone there for support. And making those big decisions related to pregnancy and birth alone can be a lot of pressure. At times, I wished I had someone to help me decide on birth plans and prenatal testing, although it also meant I had full autonomy and didn't have to make any compromises.

I wanted to tell people I was pregnant. I felt it only fair that if I expected them to support me in another loss, they should experience some love for this baby first. But I said in hushed tones, "I'm pregnant," worried I'd create bad luck if I spoke too loudly. The news was met with hugs and cheers, but I felt uncomfortable celebrating. I was already expecting the worst. I know I was happy. I do remember moments of utter contentment but the overwhelming emotion I can recall now is anxiety.

My local early pregnancy unit (EPU) said I could attend an early scan from six weeks, but my anxiety was so bad, I couldn't bring myself to make an appointment. I knew I'd be getting bad news. How could it be anything else? I'd been pregnant six times before and every time my baby had died. My body just couldn't grow babies, so, it was easier if I just lived in ignorant bliss. The longer I didn't go for the scan, the longer I could convince myself I was still pregnant. But every day got harder as I struggled with the question: Is my baby still alive or not?

Just before eight weeks, I forced myself into EPU and promptly cried on the nurse, and she kindly squeezed me in. I saw a little flickering heartbeat and sobbed again. I wasn't allowed a photo. (I have helped change the policy on this since!). But I begged the sonographer if I could take a picture on my phone. "This may be the only time I ever get to see this baby," I said through my tears, and she took pity on me and obliged.

Somehow, I got through the next two weeks and another scan. This is the furthest any pregnancy had got, and I prepared for bad news again. This time, I could see limbs wriggling about and a steady heartbeat. I was overjoyed.

I managed to get through each day, but it was a constant battle to keep my anxiety manageable. Here are some things that helped me through the tough times:

- focus on small milestones – in the beginning, this was simply getting through each day until I'd focus on getting the next scan
- I'd wake up and say: "Today I am pregnant. Whatever

happens in the future, today, here and now, I am pregnant!"
- I used to worry that my worrying about miscarrying would bring on a miscarriage. I knew this couldn't actually happen, but it's amazing how your mind spins out of control convincing you what's real. So, I'd say to myself, "It's OK to worry. Worrying or not worrying won't change the outcome."
- I gave myself permission to be anxious which then made me less anxious in the long run. I bought myself a small baby toy as a token of hope.
- getting outside in nature for walks or sitting in a park really helped me heal.

As I was doing all this on my own, in some ways it was easier as I became more selfish. If I wanted to go to bed at 6 p.m. to make the day go more quickly, then, I didn't have to worry about discussing it with my partner. I didn't have to agree with someone else about scan dates. I could just drop what I was doing and go when it suited me.

Slowly and steadily the weeks went by, but the anxiety remained ever-present. I learnt to become friends with it rather than fight it. I allowed it space, and in turn, it gave me space.

Something that surprised me when I was finally in the late stages of pregnancy was experiencing the same emotions I found difficult after loss – the baby announcements, baby showers, maternity mannequins in shops and adverts for NCT classes meant my heart rate would rise, and my chest would tighten. I'd feel jealousy, anger and guilt even though I was finally carrying my much longed-for baby. But I learnt that those emotions were all just masking sadness, for the babies I wouldn't get to hold and the pregnancy joy I'd been robbed of. Understanding that sadness was at the heart of those emotions, made it much easier to forgive myself when jealousy reared its ugly head.

Five years after deciding to go solo, four years after my first loss and then five more losses, I finally gave birth and got to hold one of my babies safely in my arms. It was only then that I could breathe easily again.

Anxiety comes in different disguises in this parenting life but I'm learning to recognise it. I say, "You're welcome, but you can't stay." Nowadays, there's only boundless room for joy.

@me_becomes_we

The truth is, you never relax

It took me and my husband nearly six years to become parents with a lot of heartache along the way. So many times, I asked, "Could this actually be our time? Or would it end in the first trimester like all the others?"

Reflecting on that first six weeks, I had some spotting and fear set in. After a blood test, I was told my HCG levels were normal, but we weren't convinced. Then my husband and I saw the tiniest little dot on the scan, a strong heartbeat, and everything was where it should be. I burst into tears. After five years, this was the first time we'd ever seen a heartbeat. It felt like a dream.

Pregnancy after loss is another journey in itself, and so is pregnancy after years of infertility. We couldn't believe it was happening, so I wouldn't allow myself to be happy or get too excited in the early days. I kept pushing the goalpost saying when we get to such and such week I can relax, but the truth is I don't think you ever relax until you bring your baby home. Even then someone told me I wouldn't relax until my child was an adult and had flown the nest.

We must have had over ten scans – the most photographed baby before he/she was even born, I'm sure. We just needed that reassurance to know our baby was healthy. The weeks went by slowly but feeling him kick as my bump grew – we found out we were having a boy – gave me so much more reassurance. Although throughout the entire pregnancy, every time I wiped, I checked for spotting; every twinge I felt made me nervous – but even if I didn't have any twinges, I'd panic too. However, I decided to enjoy the pregnancy as much as I could. It might be our only baby and I didn't want to look back and remember how scared and miserable I was.

But I was proud of my body after everything it had been through to get here. The fear never went, but as the weeks got closer to meeting him, it did get a little easier, and then right at the end when I just wanted him here safely, I panicked again.

Finally, after five and a half years of trying to conceive, four cycles of IVF, and three losses, we welcomed our baby boy in May 2021. We couldn't believe it. Our fourth IVF transfer had worked.

Many other pregnant women who haven't had the same experiences of infertility or baby loss never really understood how anxious I was, and it made me feel like I was being weird talking about it. But your feelings are always valid, and you're allowed to go through your pregnancy in whatever way makes you feel comfortable.

My advice to anyone who's experienced baby loss would be to embrace every moment. Looking back, I miss my bump. So, don't compare your pregnancy journey to anyone else's. We're all unique and have been through a different journey to get our miracles. It's ok to be anxious and excited at the same time.

Lastly, if you're reading this and are pregnant with your rainbow baby. Congratulations!

Katy Jenkins @ivf__got__this__uk and @thejstartshere

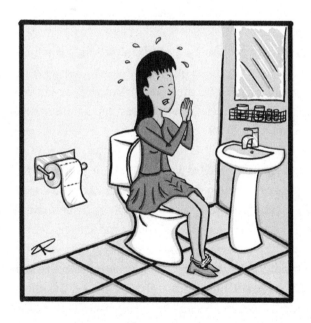

Praying at each toilet visit

It was a roller-coaster of emotions

I've spent so much time over the last ten years desperately trying to get pregnant. Unfortunately, it wasn't an easy road and I've experienced seven losses at various stages, some requiring surgical intervention. Each one was heart-breaking.

However, with each loss, my determination to continue grew stronger. My short-lived pregnancies had filled me with hope and given me a glimpse of what I'd dreamed of. I had to keep going, believing that if I could get pregnant again, it would heal some of my pain.

What I wasn't prepared for was seeing those longed for two lines on a pregnancy test again. I felt more stressed and anxious than ever. I wanted this pregnancy so badly but the fear of losing another baby consumed my thoughts and actions.

Unfortunately, I didn't have the easiest of starts to the pregnancy. I had spotting and sometimes heavier bleeding every week for up to nine weeks. I'd go to the toilet constantly to check for signs of more bleeding and I'd be devastated if there was any sign of blood. I became a regular visitor to our local EPU (Early Pregnancy Unit) who were incredibly supportive and were happy to do scans every few days to reassure me. All was well, but this made it even more of a roller-coaster of emotions.

As I progressed, any little twinge or cramp would have me googling early pregnancy symptoms. I was scared to tell people our news in case it all went wrong. I couldn't bring myself to buy anything, make plans or enjoy it as I'd hoped.

Pregnancy wasn't at all the joyful experience I thought it would be. This was something I had wished for, for so long and had day dreamed about, but the reality was very different. I guess I thought getting pregnant again would make everything better and hadn't expected the trauma and grief of the past to come back and haunt me.

Thankfully as I got to my third trimester, I felt less anxious. And by the time I had a noticeable bump and could feel the baby kicking and squirming around, I breathed a sigh of relief and tried to enjoy those magical moments of happiness.

To anyone that can relate to this, I send my love. I know it can be tough as well as heart-breaking when pregnancy isn't what you expect. I've learned that it's important to be kind to yourself, and accept that it's OK if things aren't how you imagine. Most important is aiming to find joy where you can.

Karen Hanson @aurafertility

You take everything one step at a time and with great caution

Finally, it's our turn to be pregnant and our turn to tell people that we're expecting – to feel that excitement and think ahead to the family we always dreamed of. In reality, finally becoming pregnant after five years of infertility, a pregnancy loss and four rounds of IVF didn't feel as exciting as I expected it to.

I didn't get that amazing moment of waiting to see if I had two pink lines on a pregnancy test. I didn't feel that anticipation, because I didn't even get to do a pregnancy test. I was told casually by a doctor in hospital that my blood test showed a positive pregnancy result after I was admitted with Ovarian Hyperstimulation Syndrome (OHSS). I felt so unwell and when she told me, I was alone, and I just sat on the bed and cried. My husband had gone home to get some of my things for my hospital stay, so I waited until he came back to tell him. He had much the same reaction that I did – a sigh of relief and a reserved response. We were happy of course. It was a positive first step that we'd never had before after IVF, but when you've suffered a pregnancy loss, you dare not get too excited. You take everything one step at a time and with great caution.

When we told our parents and close family, they all responded with caution, too. "That's a good first step," most of them said. There was no jumping around with tears of joy. When your family watch you go through the pain of infertility, pregnancy loss and repeated failed cycles of IVF, they've shared that pain with you.

Every small hurdle overcome was a step closer to creating our family. Every blood test result with hCG levels going in the right direction, every scan at eight weeks, ten weeks, twelve weeks showing a healthy heartbeat and our baby growing well was a small triumph. We always said to each other that we'd allow ourselves to celebrate for just that day, enjoy that happy feeling, but we couldn't get carried away. We had to stay grounded just in case.

I had the symptoms of OHSS for sixteen weeks which was tough. It prevented me from enjoying that time in my pregnancy because of the severity of the symptoms. I was so relieved when they subsided. Unfortunately, even then I didn't enjoy much of my pregnancy. I had complications with placenta previa that started when I was seventeen weeks, almost immediately after the OHSS symptoms disappeared. That was when I had my first bleed which continued on and off until the night Georgia was born at thirty-seven weeks. With every bleed came an anxiety like nothing before. I knew that if it was a small amount of blood that both myself and my baby would still be okay. However, placenta previa is unpredictable and you never know when you might have a bigger bleed that puts your baby's life in danger and possibly your own.

My husband and my family went on that roller-coaster of emotion with me after every bleed and hospital stay. Some of my close family found it hard to even talk about my baby. There wasn't much discussion about what was to come after the baby was born. There wasn't much planning or talk about baby names or decorating her nursery. It felt like everyone was holding their breath. It was hurtful at times. Sometimes it seemed like they just weren't that interested, but in reality, they were just as afraid as I was. I can see that now. It wasn't just difficult for me, it was difficult for everyone around me, too.

Every bleed with placenta previa was relatively small and settled after a few days, apart from the final bleed I experienced. I'd planned to get up at 7 a.m., as I was on the list for a caesarean that day. However, I awoke at 4 a.m. with a heavy bleed, only this time was different from the ones before. The blood loss was immense, and my husband and I were terrified.

I was rushed to hospital in an ambulance and prepped for theatre. Upon arrival, I had a trace put on which picked up Georgia's heartbeat immediately. The relief was enormous. I honestly thought I'd lost her at that stage as I couldn't fathom losing that much blood and her still being okay. She was born thirty minutes after we arrived. All those emotions I didn't dare feel while I was pregnant came flooding in – pure joy and love like nothing I'd experienced before. It was a long journey, but it was worth it when I held Georgia in my arms for the first time. She was healthy and just perfect.

Unfortunately, pregnancy with complications isn't easy; neither is being pregnant after going through fertility treatment. And it's certainly not easy after experiencing pregnancy loss. Our daughter is the light of our life, and all the happiness she brings us now, certainly makes up for what we missed when I was pregnant. Pregnancy after loss may not be what you always dreamed of and it may be filled with fear, but the joy that comes with parenthood is more than you could ever imagine. Even on the hardest days, I feel incredibly grateful to be a mother and to have Georgia as my daughter.

Suzanne Minnis @the_baby_gaim

Do I belong?

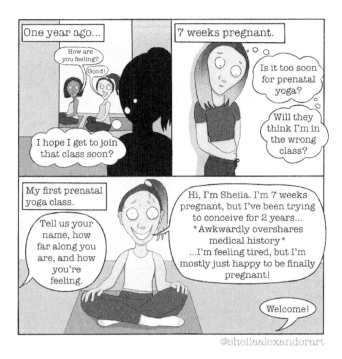

Finding out where you belong can feel difficult

It's such a blessing but also very challenging

Being pregnant after infertility and loss was a blessing but also very challenging. I was already automatically tagged as high risk which of course put pressure on me to ensure I was doing everything to keep both me and my baby safe. Going through a previous loss, I hated my body and felt it wasn't a safe space to carry a baby. However, as the pregnancy progressed, I began to trust that my body must be a safe place. When I experienced cramping and bleeding, I became afraid of what my body was doing and wished that people normalised that.

During the beginning of my first trimester, I experienced some bleeding around nine weeks and hoped it wasn't a sign of a miscarriage. I was told to come in for a scan to put my mind at ease. Sure enough, everything was fine. As the pregnancy progressed, I experienced severe cramping again and I was confused as not many mothers talked about having cramps and round ligament pain during their pregnancy. I felt that round ligament pain triggered me into thinking my body always had a problem, due to knee complications I had as a kid that required two major knee surgeries, so, I wish people were more understanding of how painful it was for me. Yes, I was seeing a chiropractor and I understood that getting treated could help the pain subside. However, having ligament issues before the pregnancy, my emotion intensified.

I was able to incorporate some coping mechanisms. I practiced being present by listening to my favorite meditation podcast series by Chel Hamilton. Walking was also a great way for me to be in touch with nature and that was the time I had to really reflect. Journaling helped me gather my thoughts and explore mantras that helped me work through my anxiety and understand how I deserved to be a mother. Writing as a Bump Day Blogger through 'Pregnancy After Loss Support' brought me peace and comfort.

I reminded myself constantly how much I'd prayed for this moment! I told myself all the reasons why I wanted to be a mother and even chose a specific song to play every morning to help me feel connected to our rainbow baby. It's called 'A New day has come' by Celine Dion. That song made me realize, I was living my truth.

Jasmine Simmons @glowful.path

My account of pregnancy after loss

From the blog: Pregnancy after loss

5th January 2019

I swing my legs into my sister's car and place my handbag at my feet.

"How are you?" she asks.

"I think I'm pregnant."

A beat passes. "Why do you think that?"

"Well, my period is late, so I took a test just now and it's positive."

"Right..."

It's Friday night and we're on our way to meet our mum and our Aunty for dinner.

"So, yeah, I guess I am pregnant. For now."

I rub at the fabric of my jeans. They are buttoned up just fine. They don't feel tight. I'm not bloated. And yet, I'm pregnant. It's good news. The best news.

The reason for the less-than-jubilant response from my sister is that I'd had a miscarriage seven months ago. I was pregnant and the baby just ceased to exist. Before that I was infertile. I say that because we didn't conceive 'naturally' after two years of trying, so that's the definition. My first daughter was conceived through IVF after many tests, lots of waiting and wondering, and much heartache. So, my current early pregnant state is fraught with trepidation.

"I feel like I'm about to get my period," I say to Cait. "Like it'll just come, and I'll do another test and the line will be fainter. And then in a few days it'll be negative."

Cait is quiet. She just listens.

"I want to be happy. But I don't dare be."

"Give it a few days."

I nod and place a hand on my lower abdomen. It's cramping with period-like pain. After two and half years of trying to conceive, I thought I could accurately analyse my body. Turns out I'm just as clueless as ever.

"Are you going to tell Mum and Aunty Linda?"

"Not sure."

In the restaurant, my Mum is having a night off. My dad has dementia and she's fast becoming his carer. It's a difficult time and we're trying to provide some light relief with our 'girl's night'. She talks us through the latest developments from the dementia support groups they're part of, options for respite care or care workers going in during the day while he's home alone, so she can carry on working. It's hard to listen to, but she's in good spirits so we go along with it and try to pretend it's not as gut wrenching as it actually is.

Then we read our menus and the inevitable conversation about sharing a bottle of wine comes up.

"Do you prefer red or white?" Aunty Linda asks me and Cait.

"I'm driving," Cait says. "I'll just have a coke."

Aunty Linda looks at me, waiting for a response. "I, uh, well, I'd probably have red to go with the pizza, but actually, I think I'll just get a coke, too."

Cait makes a show of studying her menu.

"You okay, love?" my mum asks.

"Yeah, I'm just not drinking."

I see the penny drop, almost hear it click into place.

"Oh!" she says. "Is it...are you?"

I nod.

She half leaps out of her seat then reigns herself in and sits back down, but opts for stretching across the table to take my hand and awkwardly kisses my cheek.

"What? You're what?" Aunty Linda asks, looking at us each in turn.

"I'm pregnant." I say quietly. "But it's very early and after last time ... I'm well ... I'm worried."

Aunty Linda nods. "Of course. Lovely news though. When did you find out?"

"About an hour ago."

"Oh, right. Very early then!"

"Yeah, I'll be four weeks. I'll do another test in the morning to check."

I'm jittery. I'm elated and terrified. This could be real. I might have another baby in eight months. But what if it's not real? Or what if it is real but I've already damaged the baby? I had a gin and tonic last night. I had several drinks on New Year's Eve and over Christmas. I've already worked out that I must have conceived either the night before or the night after my work Christmas do, so I'd potentially been drinking then, too. My stomach cramps again and then twists with anxiety.

"Ladies!" The waiter arrives at our table. A man who cannot read a room. "Are we celebrating tonight?"

"No," I say quickly. "Just a girl's night out."

"Great. Well, what'll it be? Champagne? Prosecco? Nice bottle of red?"

"I'll have a diet Coke please," Cait says.

"Me too," I say.

"Come on! It's Friday night! You're young! Let your hair down."

"I'm driving," Cait gives him her best polite smile.

"I just fancy a Coke."

He does an exaggerated eye roll and writes our orders down on his pad.

"Just going to the loo," I say, when he's gone.

I sit down on the closed lid and take some deep breaths. I could get my period in the morning and if I hadn't taken a test I'd never have known. I'm pregnant right now, but I know only too well that doesn't mean I'll stay that way. I think back to my first pregnancy. The elation at seeing a positive pregnancy test for the first time in my life. I didn't stop to consider then that a positive test doesn't necessarily equal a baby. I was lucky then.

At the end of the night, we go our separate ways outside the restaurant.

"Congratulations, love," my Aunty says in my ear as she gives me a tight squeeze.

I well up with tears. She's right. Whatever happens next,

congratulations are in order right now, in this moment. I smile and squeeze her back.

6th January 2019 6.19am

I squint at the clock on my bedside table. Craig is fast asleep next to me. It's pitch-black outside and the heating has only just clicked on, so it's still cold as I swing my legs out of bed and pad to the bathroom. I have three pregnancy tests waiting. All different brands. I open them and wee on them all at the same time. I don't have to wait long. Two pink lines, a blue cross, the word 'Pregnant' on a digital display. I breathe a little.

25th January 2019

The bottle of water they've given me to drink is ice cold and it's chilly in the waiting room. I can't stop shivering. Whether it's purely from the temperature is difficult to say. We're waiting for our 'reassurance scan' at a private clinic. The NHS wouldn't scan me early because there's no medical reason to do so, despite my lovely GP doing her best to ask. It's okay. I didn't really want to go back to the early pregnancy unit in the hospital where I'd been after my miscarriage. Bad memories. Here they sell photo frames for your scan photos, teddy bears, gender reveal balloons. The floors are wooden, the walls white. There are plants and fish tanks. It feels expensive.

I've made it this far. Pregnancy tests are still very definitely positive (yes, I'm still doing them), and my period didn't come the next day or the day after that. And the cramping stopped. I should be around seven weeks pregnant.

"Tori Day?"

A young, dark-haired woman pokes her head out of the only door.

I stand up and Craig follows. The room through the door is similar to a scanning room in a hospital, but it smells different. Instead of disinfectant, it's incense. Imagine BUPA clinic meets yoga retreat, and you wouldn't be too far off.

"Come and lay down here." The woman pats the bed. I do as I'm told.

"Are you okay? You're shaking."

"Just cold."

"Yes, sorry about that. Takes a while to warm up in here and I'm afraid this gel is going to be cold on your tummy as well."

"Oh, is it not a dildo cam? Erm, sorry," I cough. "I mean an internal scan?"

"No, we're not medically trained. But if you're seven weeks, we should be able to see from the outside."

I don't like the word 'should'. But what can I do? Demand she insert a probe into my vagina? Not socially acceptable. Leave? Not a chance.

My shaking ramps up and I try to think warm thoughts. I breathe deeply and will my body to stay still. The gel goes on. The wand moves over my stomach. The woman squints at the grainy screen. I can't breathe. I close my eyes. It's quiet. The wand is still moving.

"I'm afraid..." My stomach drops through the bed, the floor, and to the centre of the earth. "I can't get a good enough look. Your bladder isn't full enough. I'm really sorry, but I'm going to need you to drink some more water and give it twenty minutes or so."

My body is rigid with the effort of trying to stop shaking.

"Come on, it's okay." Craig has hold of my hand. "Finish this and we'll come back in."

He hands me the ice-cold water and we go back to the waiting area.

It's not bad news, it's no news, I tell myself as I look at the teddy bears, the fish, the balloons. What if she couldn't see it because there's nothing to see? No, stop it! Stop it!

"Not long now," Craig says.

The woman calls us back in. I close my eyes again. Hold my breath.

"That's better. I've got a nice clear view now. And here's something ... yes, here's the heartbeat."

I open my eyes. There's a grainy flicker on the screen.

"Are you sure?" I ask.

"Yes." She smiles and points to the flicker. Craig is squeezing my hand.

A sound that is a half-laugh, half-cry bursts out of me. The shaking stops. Tears slide down my face and wet the pillow under my head.

"Oh," is all I can manage.

"Can you tell how far along?" Craig asks.

I'm grateful one of us is able to string a sentence together.

"Seven weeks, one day. Estimated due date: 10th September."

The tears come thick and fast now. I can breathe for the first time in three weeks.

"Are you okay?" the woman asks for the second time that morning.

"Yes, I just … I had a miscarriage previously, and my first baby was conceived through IVF, so I can't quite believe this is happening.'

She smiles.

"It's happening. Would you like some photos?"

Tori Day @toridaywarrior

Link to blog: https://toridayblog.wordpress.com

I prepared my heart for another loss

I remember being fourteen very well. I'd already been menstruating for four years, and by that time I was familiar with annual pap smears. I'd already had one fibroid surgically removed and was on the birth control pill to control my ovarian cysts and regulate my cycle. The visit to my OB/GYN was different, though, because that year, I had a boyfriend, and he had a car with a big backseat.

"Getting pregnant is so easy," my OB/GYN said as he sat down at his desk to give me the 'talk'. "You can get pregnant through jeans!"

"Um, what?" I said with a squeaky voice.

"Yep! You can get pregnant through jeans. You can get pregnant sitting on a toilet if there's sperm on it. Sperm is very powerful. Are you prepared to raise a baby?" he asked with a smirk.

Panic set in and as I wondered if I needed a pregnancy test, he said, "Okay, maybe, it's not that powerful, but your Mom told me to scare you enough so you wouldn't have sex!"

I left that appointment and every appointment thereafter for the next five years terrified I'd get pregnant, because "sperm is that powerful!". And I didn't have much to say to my Mom on the way home either. I already resented my body for menstruating so early and now I was terrified that my period would lead to pregnancy, and I wasn't ready to raise a baby.

I never considered women couldn't get pregnant or miscarried their babies. So, when I was nineteen and had my first miscarriage, I was heartbroken. Two years later, I miscarried my second baby, and I was never the same again. I spent my twenties convincing myself I didn't want children. It hurt too much. Since I'd gotten pregnant previously while on the pill, I made sure to take extra precautions.

Flash forward to my thirties and I was now married to the man of my dreams, and we wanted 'our baby'. My husband had mended my heart and I felt whole enough to build a family. But after two years of trying, we were unable to conceive and started our IVF journey.

Faith was conceived by IVF and I convinced myself that the embryo transfer wouldn't work. I wanted a baby. We wanted our baby. But now I was scared to be pregnant and at the same time, I was fearful of never being pregnant.

I was so concerned that when the doctor called to tell me I was pregnant, I didn't believe her. After reality kicked in, I instinctively prepared for another loss, thinking things like: "I'll be devastated. I'm not meant to have children of my own." My pregnancy was complicated. So, on the hour, I'd check for signs of a miscarriage. Any twinge or cramp would send me running to the bathroom. At one point I was told that Faith may not survive childbirth. So even when I was in labor, I was still mentally preparing myself for heartbreak.

When Faith was finally handed to me by the NICU Doctor, she scored a nine out of ten on the Apgar scale. The panic, the fear, the anxiety didn't stop until she was placed into my arms and nuzzled close. That's the moment when I accepted the love and joy that comes with having a baby. This is pregnancy after loss! This intense fear that something will happen to your baby despite your brain convincing you that "it'll be okay".

I've now lost six babies to miscarriage. After my last loss, two years ago, I was sure there were no more tears to cry, but I've learned that grief is acceptable and necessary. I miss my daughter's heartbeat and her kicks, but through grief, I realized that I'm still the mother to all of my babies, and they'll forever be my babies.

Grief doesn't go away. It's not something you 'get over'. But somehow we learn to live with that pain, and even thrive, despite it. But that emotion is different for everyone. We all have our own stories, and we all experience things differently. I picture grief as the ocean. We learn to walk through the ocean but, once in a while, a wave swells and knocks us down, perhaps even pulls us under, briefly, but we manage to clamber up and find out way back to shore. That's where you'll find me, on the shore.

Annette Pearson @thatwarriorannette

I felt naked without my infertility label

Five months after moving to a new country with a new partner, and getting a new job teaching music, I was finally pregnant. I was also surrounded by other expectant mothers that were juggling teaching and pregnancy better than me. And no doubt conceived quicker than I did. Strangely, I felt naked without my infertility label. In one sense it was freeing to start over and not have the weight of that label, but in another sense, it was part of my identity for ten years. How do you live without it?

I wasn't sure how to talk about my infertility story to new people. It was a painful wound I didn't always want to expose. Some assumed that because my partner and I had been together such a short time – although we'd known each other for years – that this was an accident. That hurt me. I didn't want anyone assuming that this child I'd desperately waited for, wasn't conceived on purpose. It made me want to hide my growing belly.

I wanted to wait as long as possible before telling my students I was pregnant, but on my rough days when I was exhausted and having trouble making music or even singing, I desperately wanted to say something, just so they might be kinder to me.

But the longer I said nothing, the longer I wanted to keep it a secret. That was partly because I wasn't sure how to tell people, and partly because I wasn't ready to open myself up to all the criticism that comes with both infertility and pregnancy.

I'd return home from work and often spend the afternoon resting. I thought I'd want to write in my journal, but I hardly wrote anything. Instead, I saved all my energy for creating my child. And in my moments alone, I'd feel the wonder of this baby growing inside me.

At sixteen weeks pregnant, I had a horrible pain but instinctively, I felt everything would be OK. Sitting in the emergency room surrounded by lots of other struggling pregnant women was probably the worst part. It was like a squirmy mass of big bellies and unspoken fears hovering amongst us. I wasn't worried about losing my baby because I could feel movement in my belly, but I was worried about how I was going to survive this pregnancy. I felt broken. Why couldn't I just have a normal, healthy pregnancy after everything I'd already been through?

When they did the ultrasound, they discovered the reason for the pain was that I had multiple fibroids (non-cancerous tumors) in my uterus. The largest was 11 x 5 x 7cm.

At the twenty-week ultrasound, they finally measured the baby instead of the fibroids. When they explained we had a perfectly healthy baby, I started weeping. That was the turning point where I truly started to believe I would hold my baby in my arms. Before that, I still avoided going to any baby stores and would feel physically sick at the thought. But I gave myself permission to find some second-hand clothes and furniture through groups online.

Through the hardest moments of the pregnancy and the birth process, music was something that carried me onward. When I struggled, singing a song would help me through. Shortly after my child was birthed, a song I had written came up on my playlist. That song is about taking risks in life and that God will be with you along your journey. My joy was seeing my child laying on my chest, simply breathing in life together, making the journey so worth it.

Leah Irby @leahirby

Thank you for buying this book

It means a lot to all of us who have put this book together that we are helping and supporting you, and raising awareness outside of the TTC (trying to conceive) community.

We would all love to help more people but there are only a handful of us, and lots of you. Would you help spread the word that this book can support those on this roller-coaster journey to parenthood? It's very easy and will take you a minute. You can:

- share the book on your social media accounts
- if you support pregnant clients let them know that this book is a great resource
- leave a review or rating on the site you downloaded/bought it from
- leave a review on Goodreads
- send me your review and I'll gladly share it on social media
- let influential people in your community know that the book can help their followers
- tell healthcare professionals who you work with, and/or who support you, that the book is available and can help their other clients, and raise awareness.

I am very passionate about raising awareness of how common infertility and loss is, and the emotional realities of this journey. I'm hopeful that by sharing our stories there will eventually be no stigma or shame associated with these topics, which means future generations will feel supported and not alone. If you would like to help raise awareness, why don't you gift a paperback copy to a family member or friend, especially if you want them to know what you're going through but find it difficult to explain. If you're a professional working in your own practice and would like to gift the paperback to your clients or have the eBook available on your website for your clients to download, please contact me at the above email address for bulk discount or eBook subscription rates.

If you have a podcast or need guest posts for your website or blog site, I am always happy to share my story so that it may help others. Please see my website: www.mfsbooks.com for more information about all my books. I make a small donation from this sale to an appropriate charity in your country.

Wishing you all the very best on your journey to meet your baby.

Love Sheila xxx

Other Fertility Books

Please visit my website www.mfsbooks.com or Instagram @fertilitybooks for more information.

FREE eBook: The Best Fertility Jargon Buster: The most concise A-Z list of fertility abbreviations and acronyms you will ever need
Are you confused by the infertility abbreviations used on social media sites? It's like a new language you need to learn at a very stressful time, isn't it? This book is your must-have companion - a comprehensive list of over 250 need-to-know medical and non-medical abbreviations and acronyms, to help you as you navigate this roller-coaster journey.

Sign up to download the FREE eBook here and join my newsletter: www.mfsbooks.co.uk

This is Trying To Conceive: Real-life experiences from the TTC community
Infertility sucks doesn't it? Do you feel that no one understands what this is like, and you've had enough of the insensitive, unhelpful comments? Read over thirty true-life stories from the fabulous TTC community, who want to support you and let you know that you are not alone.

Available to download as a FREE eBook here: www.mfsbooks.com/free-ebook and in print here: https://books2read.c

om/u/bPXw27

This is IVF and Other Fertility Treatments: Real-life experiences of going through fertility treatments

Have you recently found out you'll need fertility treatment to get pregnant? Are you currently preparing for an IVF (in-vitro fertilization) cycle? Or maybe you've done other unsuccessful treatments, and you've now decided to move to IVF. Read over thirty honest, emotional short stories from infertility warriors, about what it's really like to do fertility treatment. They have your back and are here whenever you need them, day or night.

Available in print and as an eBook here; https://books2read.c om/u/31YVp6

This is the Two Week Wait: Real-life experiences of the IVF and assisted fertility treatment two-week wait

Does the thought of the two-week wait fill you with dread? Would you like some company until it's test day? Read other women's stories and experiences of how they navigated this 'wait' and arrived at test day in one piece.

Available in print and as an eBook here: https://books2read.c om/u/47YV1j

This is Pregnancy and Baby Loss: Real-life experiences from the baby loss community

Have you experienced pregnancy or baby loss recently, or in the past? Do you feel alone, and that no one understands you are grieving? If this is you, I am so very sorry for your loss. Other baby loss parents share their honest stories in this book – early and late pregnancy loss, ectopic pregnancy, recurrent pregnancy loss, the loss of a twin, and stillbirth. They understand your pain and offer support and comfort on each page.

Available in print and as an eBook here: https://books2read.com/u/bQdAL7

Infertility Doesn't Care About Ethnicity: Encouraging tales about conception struggles

The emotions we feel when it's challenging to conceive are the same for all women, but women from ethnic communities often face additional pressure from their culture, community, the medical profession and social media. Encouraging tales about conception struggles - including IVF, pregnancy and baby loss, donor conception, surrogacy and childfree after infertility - will offer you the support and validation you deserve.

Available as a FREE eBook here: www.mfsbooks.com/infertility-doesnt-care/ Also available in print.

My Fertility Book; All the fertility and infertility explanations you will ever need, from A to Z

Are you stressed navigating the world of conception? Do you feel overwhelmed by the sheer amount of infertility information available online? This comprehensive, jargon-free book explains over 200+ medical and non-medical terms and includes helpful illustrations. Available in print and as an eBook here: https://books2read. com/u/mq0Nd2

Resources

Below are the biographies and contact details for the contributors who wanted to be listed in case you would like to connect with them. If what they have written resonates with you, I'm sure they would love to hear from you, and please tell them you read their story in this book!

Alex Kornswiet is a blogger at 'Our Beautiful Surprise', where she talks openly about her journey to motherhood, infertility, pregnancy loss, pregnancy, and motherhood. The community is very active on Instagram where it raises awareness and offers support for infertility, pregnancy loss, and parenting after these traumas.

If you would like to connect with Alex:
Instagram @ourbeautifulsurprise
Website https://www.ourbeautifulsurprise.com/
Email alex.ourbeautifulsurprise@gmail.com

Alyssa Madrid resides in San Francisco with her husband, Steven, and puppy, Bailey. They've been trying to conceive since 2018. Alyssa is passionate about all thing's fertility and health, which is what moved her to start her Instagram account. It's given her a space to openly and honestly share her journey with infertility, IVF, and loss. The community has brought much comfort and Alyssa hopes that by sharing her story she can empower other women to do the same.

If you would like to connect with Alyssa:

Instagram @healthivf

Annette Pearson is a wife to Tom, a mother to Faith, a bonus mother to Jonathan and Bailey and a mother to her six heavenly babies. After her daughter was born asleep in January 2020, she attended a support group and shared her story, and now pays that support forward by helping other women through her blog and on her social media. She's an author and published her first book, *Finding Strength in the Dark*, in January 2021; her memoir that she hopes will help women to find their strength too.

If you would like to connect with Annette:

Instagram @thatwarriorannette

Arden Cartrette is a Certified Birth & Bereavement Doula and a trauma response specialist had her own infertility journey that included two first trimester births before giving birth to her and her husband's son, Cameron, in February 2020. Having made it through the thick of grief and pregnancy after loss, she knew that it was time to create a space where women are able to get the support that she never had. So she founded The Miscarriage Doula in 2020 which is a place for every woman who feels alone in her miscarriage journey.

If you would like to connect with Arden:

Instagram @themiscarriagedoula

Website https://www.themiscarriagedoula.co/

Christina Oberon is the author of *Hope Strong: Navigating the Emotions of Your Infertility Journey: Overcome the Pain and Thrive with Hope* and children's book, *Embaby Elio*. She lives in

Southern California with her husband, Kevin, and son, Kai. She enjoys traveling, advocating for worthy causes, supporting the infertility community and has a passion for health and wellness.

If you would like to connect with Christina:

Instagram @xtina.o_

Clare is a DEIVF (IVF donor egg) mama to a baby girl born March 2022, a trainee nutritionist and infertility veteran. Her six-year infertility 'journey' included six miscarriages, five fertility clinics, an ectopic pregnancy ending in surgery, and too many injections, medications, egg collections and embryo transfers! She says: "What I have found throughout our long and often painful fertility journey is that, as well as the many lows there have also been incredible positives, and I genuinely believe this experience has changed my life for the better, as I have found out how strong I am and I have found my passion and purpose in life, and that is nutrition. Most of all though, at the end of this long and shi**y road, I have the baby girl I was always meant to have, and I wouldn't change her for the world!"

If you would like to connect with Clare:

Instagram @iwannabeamamabear

Crystal-Gayle and Miguel Williams founded 4Damani in October 2018 after experiencing the death of their first child Damani, in the September. After recognizing how unmentionable baby loss and grief are in Jamaica, coupled with the lack of support, the cause was established to acknowledge and support grieving parents. The aim of 4Damani is to break the silence and stigma surrounding pregnancy and infant loss in Jamaica by sharing stories so persons know they're not alone. Through their advocacy, in June 2019, the Governor General of Jamaica proclaimed October as Pregnancy and Infant Loss Awareness Month in Jamaica, and October 15th as Pregnancy and Infant Loss Remembrance Day. Crystal-Gayle as since given birth to Damani's sister.

If you would like to connect with Crystal-Gayle:
Instagram/Twitter/Facebook @4Damani
Website https://www.4damani.com

Erin Bulcao says; "I have been married to my husband Nick for twelve years now and we have twins, Eliana and Natalia and a one-year-old, Eriela Nicole. We conceived the twins through an IUI (because unexplained infertility/ no period), and ended up with triplets, thus forcing us to face a medical reduction at nine weeks pregnant. The trauma of that and infertility took a toll on our marriage, but we worked on it for years and then decided to try IVF for our third. After three years, four egg retrievals, a miscarriage and seven transfers, we finally got our rainbow baby. We have one mosaic embryo left and are pursuing further information on mosaicism and risks. I live in Encinitas, CA, but spend a lot of time in NYC. My husband is a born and raised San Diegan' and while I lived in Mexico City until I was 11, and still have all of my family there, SoCal has been my home. I am a devoted chocolate lover and anything musical theatre with a side of red wine. Warm regards, Erin

If you would like to connect with Erin:
Instagram @Mybeautifulblunder.com

Grace Miano went through several years trying to conceive, which included a surprise diagnosis of endometriosis and three miscarriages after natural conception. Her first IVF cycle resulted in one embryo, which went on to be her rainbow baby, who was born when Grace was forty-three. It's now her focus to become an advocate and industry leader in miscarriage and pregnancy after loss, and she's made it her mission to speak openly in an effort to smash the taboo and isolation of pregnancy loss. She is based in Melbourne, Australia, and is a Miscarriage Practitioner, Nutritionist, Womb & Fertility Massage Therapist, Miscarriage Doula, BHSci(NutMed), BA(Psych), PGradCertEd, CertTAE, CIMI.

If you'd like to connect with Grace:

Instagram @thegracemiano

Website https://www.gracemiano.com/ for her Pregnancy after loss program, Guided relaxations/meditations, and Miscarriage doula support

Book to see me www.gracemiano.com/bookings

Helene Tubridy Helena Tubridy is a fertility coach, hypnotherapist, EMDR therapist and former midwife. She believes mindset is key in natural fertility, and IVF success, along with lifestyle advice and medically accurate information. Helena helps clients after pregnancy loss, premature birth, stillbirth and birth trauma. Sessions are via Zoom. As a fertility health advocate, Helena regularly contributes on TV, radio, press and podcast.

If you would like to connect with Helena:

Instagram @helenatubridy

Website https://www.helenatubridy.com

Jasmine Simmons is an infertility and miscarriage advocate, a blogger and Mom to Jowen after three rounds of IVF.

If you would like to connect with Jasmine:

Instagram @glowful.path

Email Jevainsimmons@gmail.com

Blog https://pregnancyafterlosssupport.org/author/jasmine-simmons/

Jennifer Robertson is a fertility coach and has helped women all over the world transform their mindset and take back control of their life in the midst of infertility. She is also the author of ***The Injustice of Infertility***, a deeply inspiring and raw account of her own seven-year fertility journey. Throughout her own fertility journey, Jen discovered that her old ways of pushing and working hard weren't serving her. She is now using the lessons learned along the way to develop programs and support women throughout their journey to motherhood - from the moment they start trying to conceive, until they hold their baby in their arms.

If you would like to connect with Jennifer for fertility support:
Instagram @msjenniferrobertson
Website www.jenniferrobertson.co
Or for pregnancy after loss or infertility support:
Instagram @yourpregnancyhaven
Website www.yourpregnancyhaven.co

Karen Hanson has her own infertility and loss story and is the co-founder of Aura Fertility. Aura is an evidence-based emotional support app, developed with experts to provide whole-person well-being support during fertility treatment, helping people to feel supported through the ups and downs at every turn of the journey.

If you would like to connect with Karen:
Instagram @aurafertility
Website www.aura-fertility.com

Kate Knapton says "I'm a wife and mama to two sweet kids. We have MFI (male factor infertility) and were given less than .02% chance of having genetic children. We decided to pursue embryo donation adoption and we received six embryos from our donors. We have experienced three chemical pregnancies and still have three embryos remaining. I am a stay-at-home mama and create and sell jewelry for those experiencing infertility."

If you would like to connect with Kate:

Instagram @jojiiandco

Email: jojiiandco@gmail.com

Website www.jojiiandco.com

Katy Jenkins is thirty years old and is married to Thomas, who's thirty-two. They live in Exeter, Devon in the UK with their fur-baby Stan. They have been TTC for five years and have experienced natural losses and failed IVF transfers. They have found social media TTC accounts extremely helpful and supportive during their journey. They decided to create a fertility sock company called 'The Journey Starts Here' with the hope that their socks will bring joy to such an incredibly hard journey. They also think it's a great way to tell your story via social media and to connect with other men and women who understand the struggles of infertility. Katy also treats them as her lucky socks too. In May 2021 after a successful fourth embryo transfer Katy gave birth to her rainbow baby boy Parker.

If you would like to connect with Katy and Tom:

Instagram @thejstartshere and @ivf_got_this_uk

Website www.the-journey-starts-here.myshopify.com

Leah Irby is the creator of *Connecting with Spirit Baby: for a courageous conception and pregnancy*, and the author of the

Gender Rainbow children's book series. She is also a recording artist and music educator who has lived in the US, India, and Sweden. She became a mom when she was forty-three.

If you would like to connect with Leah:

Instagram @leahirby

Facebook @newconceptionsbyleahirby

Online courses https://bit.ly/naturalanxietyrelief

SoundCloud @leahirby

YouTube https://bit.ly/leah-irby-YouTube

Lyndsey Clabby, a co-founder of myMindBodyBaby, a business dedicated to increasing support and empowerment for those struggling with their fertility. With over twelve years of experience in CPG and Pharmaceutical brand management and a passion for helping others, Lyndsey has helped build myMindBodyBaby from the ground up. She has a Bachelor of Medical Science in Biochemistry, an MBA from Ivey, and is a certified fitness instructor. After struggling for years with infertility, she and her husband were able to conceive their first son through their last remaining IVF embryo. Lyndsey and her husband now have three children, two sons and a daughter, and live in Mississauga, Ontario, Canada.

If you would like to connect with Lyndsey:

Instagram @mymindbodybaby

Website www.mymindbodybaby.com

Facebook @mymindbodybabypage

Pinterest @mymindbodybaby

Mark Morrison is the author of *Whirlwinds to Rainbow – the story to Us*. He and his wife Kim experienced recurring pregnancy loss before welcoming their two children, and as a grateful father, he wrote his book in order to celebrate all women who have fought or continue to fight, to get their rainbow baby.

If you would like to connect with Mark and Kim:

Instagram @bombprooffamily

Nora experienced four pregnancy losses before welcoming her daughter in to her life, and now has baby number two on the way. She is passionate about perinatal mental health and supports women going through pregnancy after loss.

If you would like to connect with Nora:

Instagram @thislimboland

Suzanne Minnis experienced three failed IVF (in vitro fertilisation) cycles that left her devastated and wondering if she would ever become a mum. On their fourth cycle, Suzanne and her husband got their BFP, (positive pregnancy test) and she is now mama to their miracle daughter. She now blogs about fertility, IVF and motherhood.

If you would like to connect with Suzanne:

Instagram @the_baby_gaim

Blog www.thebabygaim.com

Tori Day lives with her husband and two children in West Yorkshire. After struggling to get pregnant with her first daughter, she felt compelled to write about her experience of infertility and IVF with the aim of helping others. *Warrior* is Tori's personal account of battling infertility and attempting to stay sane while trying to conceive. Her second book, *The Unchosen Life*, is a fiction novel which tells the story of Clara, the woman whose infertility journey doesn't end with a baby, and how she finds happiness and fulfilment in a life she didn't choose. Both are available on Amazon.

If you would like to connect with Tori:

Instagram @ToriDayWarrior

Twitter @ToriDayWrites

Blog https://toridayblog.wordpress.com

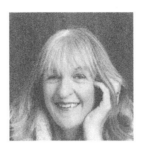

About the Author

Sheila Lamb had a six-year infertility journey involving fertility treatments, and pregnancy loss. A week after her forty-seventh birthday, she welcomed her rainbow daughter into the world, who was conceived using a donor egg. Sheila now supports others through her *Fertility Books* series. On Instagram, she's a champion for highlighting other author's books on all subjects to do with trying to conceive and loss, as she knows reading other people's stories is so helpful and comforting when the journey to parenthood is a struggle. Follow her on Instagram @fertilitybooks.

You can connect with me on:
🌐 https://www.mfsbooks.com
📘 https://facebook.com/SheilaLamb/Author

Subscribe to my newsletter:
✉ https://mfsbooks.co.uk

Printed in Great Britain
by Amazon

81001860R00081